ALSO BY JEANNE JONES

The Calculating Cook: A Gourmet Cookbook for Diabetics &
   Dieters
Diet for a Happy Heart: A Low-Cholesterol, Low-Calorie
   Cookbook
The Fabulous Fiber Cookbook: Recipes High in Fiber and Low in
   Calories
Secrets of Salt-Free Cooking: A Complete Low-Sodium Cookbook
Fitness First—A 14-Day Diet & Exercise Program
The Fabulous Fructose Recipe Book
Jeanne Jones' Party Planner and Entertaining Diary
More Calculated Cooking: Practical Recipes for Diabetics and
   Dieters
Ambition's Woman, a novel
Stuffed Spuds: 100 Meals in a Potato
The Love in the Afternoon Cookbook
Jeanne Jones' Food Lover's Diet: A Safe, Sane Way to Stay Thin
   Forever

JET FUEL

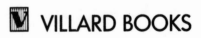

VILLARD BOOKS

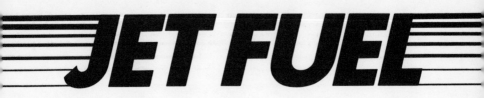

JET FUEL

The New Food Strategy for the High-Performance Person

JEANNE JONES

NEW YORK   1984

Library of Congress Cataloging in Publication Data

Jones, Jeanne.
  Jet fuel.

  1. Nutrition.   2. Diet.   I. Title.
RA784.J66   1984   613.2'8   83-21856
ISBN 0-394-53588-X

Manufactured in the United States of America
9 8 7 6 5 4 3 2
First Edition

Grateful acknowledgment is made to M. Evans & Co., Inc. for permission to reprint
the recipe from *Stuffed Spuds: 100 Meals in a Potato* by Jeanne Jones. Copyright ©
1982 by Jeanne Jones. Reprinted by permission of the publisher, M. Evans & Co.,
Inc., New York, N.Y. 10017.

A special thanks to the *Canyon Ranch Menu and Recipe Book.*

Information regarding an audio-cassette program on the *JET FUEL* concept may be
obtained from Nightingale Conant Corporation, 7300 N. Lehigh Avenue, Chicago,
Illinois 60648.

Designed by Oksana Kushnir

To Charlie—for the next hundred years!

IN GRATEFUL ACKNOWLEDGMENT:
Robert Bernstein
Robert Gros
Marc Jaffe
Spencer Johnson
Margaret McBride
Viola Stroup
Susan Wallach

Contents

1	Taking Off	1
2	Fuel Facts Calorie Density and Fuel Sources	13
3	Modern Marketing and Streamlining the Galley	39
4	*JET FUEL* in Transition From Raw Materials to Menus	47
5	*JET FUEL* in Motion In Restaurants, on Jets, Brown-Bagging, and Being a Guest	85
6	Jet Age Psychology	93

JET FUEL

Taking Off

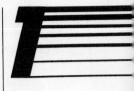

Have you ever wondered why some people never seem to have to worry about their weight or staying in shape? They are lean, fit, energetic people who can best be described as high performers. For these high-performance people, success—both socially and professionally—seems automatic. How do they manage to keep up the pace of work and exercise along with dining out frequently, going to parties, traveling, entertaining, and still remain in such fantastic shape? *Easily*—they run on *JET FUEL!*

JET FUEL is a positive food strategy—an exciting way of looking at life, an attitude of health, energy, and achievement.

Eating for success can be learned more easily than dressing for success, and will have a far greater impact on your life. Successful eating can best be described as providing the body with superior fuel so that it looks, feels, and performs at its best. Frequently we eat only what is readily available at the time, forgetting that *food is our only fuel.*

Every function of the body depends on the quality of the fuel provided. Too often we fail to remember this includes the brain and therefore the entire reasoning process. With *JET FUEL* you not only look better, feel better, and have more energy—you also think more clearly and have a greatly improved memory. You are actually smarter, because you are using more of the brain's capacity. You work more efficiently and can accomplish much more in much less time.

THE FUEL MIX

Our fuel is made up of many parts. The essential components are the three basic food groups: carbohydrates, proteins, and fats. However, all other additives to the fuel, such as water, alcohol, salt, sugar, sugar substitutes, caffeine, and condiments—whether they are beneficial or harmful—are still part of the fuel mix and affect our performance.

Ordinary fuel—high in fat, cholesterol, salt, sugar, alcohol, and caffeine—makes you fat, clogs your arteries, and raises your blood pressure. Using fat for fuel causes early burnout because of a clogged engine and keeps you from flying high or fast. Sugar in the fuel gets you airborne in a hurry but causes crash landings. Too much salt in the fuel causes so much fluid to accumulate that you may not be able to take off in the first place. Caffeine provides only false starts. Too much alcohol in the mix can keep you from landing at the right destination. Ordinary fuel is *not* for the high-performance person who doesn't want to waste time on slow starts, risky flying, or short flights.

The difference between *JET FUEL* and ordinary fuel is in the mix.

The good news is that *you* can mix *JET FUEL* yourself through your own food selection. The *secret* to *JET FUEL* is combining at least five times as much *in volume* of complex carbohydrates as animal protein. To visualize this, picture two plastic containers, one five times as large as the other. Think of putting your salad, vegetables, potatoes, rice, pasta, or bread and fruit in the large container. Then think of putting your fish, poultry, meat, or dairy products in the smaller container. The smaller container doesn't have to be full. In other words, animal protein doesn't have to constitute one-fifth of the volume of your meal. The important concept is that animal protein should never be *more than* one-fifth of your meal.

Old-fashioned, traditional menu-planning always started with "What will I serve with the roast?" *JET FUEL* menu-planning is the other way around. Think of the fish, poultry, or meat as the side dish and the salad, vegetables, breads, and pastas as the main part of the meal.

The goals of *JET FUEL* are: Increase the complex carbohydrates, decrease the animal protein, and limit the intake of fats.

The complex carbohydrates are your power source. They are the cleanest-burning fuel and provide a quick source of energy. They include all the beautiful fresh fruits and vegetables, tasty textured whole-grain breads, cereals, and pastas.

Enough protein is needed for the growth, maintenance and repair of body cells. However, protein is a slower-burning fuel and does not provide energy as quickly as carbohydrates. Complex carbohydrates and proteins, in the proper combination, provide the best sustained sources of energy. Good sources of protein include delicious fresh fish, poultry, and meat; light low-fat dairy products; and legumes.

Limiting the intake of fat reduces the buildup of grime that prevents the body from running efficiently. Fat is the slowest-burning, least efficient fuel source. Fat is also the leading source of calories. For this reason, fat will make you fat faster than anything else.

JET FUEL ———————————————————3

JET FUEL MIX

5 TIMES AS MUCH COMPLEX CARBOHYDRATES AS ANIMAL PROTEIN

6 to 8 glasses of water

COMPLEX CARBOHYDRATES

Vegetables
Fruits
Whole grain products:
    Breads
    Pasta
    Cereals

ANIMAL PROTEIN

Fish
Poultry
Lean Meat
Dairy Products

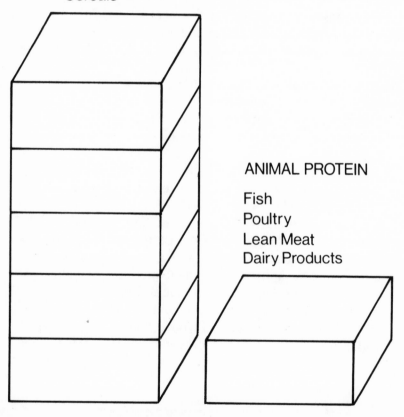

All the fat necessary for good nutrition is present in the complex carbohydrate and protein foods you eat. It is not necessary to add any extra fat to a well-balanced meal. Therefore, use fat sparingly and only for flavor and moisture. Included in the fat category are butter, margarine, oils, salad dressings, and mayonnaise, as well as high-fat cheeses, fat-marbled meat, the skin of poultry, nuts, and seeds.

The importance of drinking enough water for *JET FUEL* cannot be overstressed. Add six to eight glasses of water to the mix every day. Use salt and sugar sparingly and drink alcoholic beverages only in moderation.

You're flying on JET FUEL!

JET FUEL does *not* mean that you can eat copious quantities of food and become stronger, smarter, and slimmer as long as you combine the fuels you are using in the right ratio. In other words, it is *not* okay to eat a twelve-ounce steak as long as you balance it with five times the amount in volume of grains, vegetables, and fruit. Think instead in terms of a three- or four-ounce steak or a piece of chicken instead of half a chicken, then visualize the rest of your meal in proportion to your serving of animal protein. When you take in more fuel of any type than the body can use, it is stored as fat, potentially dangerous to your health and certainly detrimental to your appearance.

How much fuel is enough? The amount needed to support normal growth in children and desirable weight in adults. You would not overfuel an airplane. If you know that the fuel tank on your own car holds only twenty gallons, you would not put twenty-five gallons in it. It would spill out and be potentially dangerous. It is equally dangerous to overfuel your body constantly. If you need only five or six hundred calories at a meal for energy, why put in two thousand? It won't spill out, but it certainly will *bulge* out.

Many scientists believe that eating less to maintain an ideal consistent weight is the key to increasing both the length and the quality of life. Along with eating less to live longer, they emphasize the importance of significantly reducing consumption of fat and proteins that are associated with such killers as heart disease and cancer and eating more grains, vegetables, and fruits that appear to offer some protection against these diseases.

Current nutritional guidelines for the exact percentages of carbohydrates, proteins, and fats vary from one expert to another. They suggest that anywhere from 50 to 60 percent complex carbohydrates, from 10 to 20 percent proteins and from 10 to 30 percent fats should make up the total calories consumed. Realistically, no one eats by computer printouts. The guidelines all tell us the same thing—fly on *JET FUEL!*

Dr. Roy L. Walford, in his book *Maximum Life Span*, explains that the key is undernutrition, not malnutrition. Undernutrition means a reduction in total calorie intake while maintaining normal levels of important nutrients and getting down to a body weight that is several pounds lower than standard weight charts' recommendations.

Even older animals that are put on restricted diets tend to live longer. "It is therefore not too late to repent in adult life," says Dr. Hamish Nisbet Munro of the United States Department of Agriculture's Human Nutrition Research Center on Aging at Tufts University.

This new research does not suggest that people can live forever, but that they *can* reach their maximum life span in good physical and mental health. After reaching the end of this span—estimated to be well over hundred years—death would come quickly without years of chronic disease.

JET FUEL eliminates middle age!

With *JET FUEL* you don't have to give up anything you truly *enjoy. JET FUEL* offers maximum flexibility because you can eat *anything* just as long as you combine the things you like best in the right ratio. *JET FUEL* also offers you a wide variety of tastes and textures that will make your meals much more interesting.

After flying on *JET FUEL* for just a short time, your basic tastes will change quickly, and you will start choosing the ingredients for *JET FUEL* because you will really prefer them over ordinary fuel. When you use less dressing on your salad, you will start enjoying the delightful natural tastes and crunchiness of fresh fruits and vegetables more than you ever have before. A salad swimming in dressing will no longer appeal to you.

Whole-grain breads offer much more variety in taste and texture than their refined white counterparts. After being spoiled by the many choices available in whole-grain products, you will find white breads boring by comparison. Also, using less butter or margarine on your toast will give you a new appreciation of the wonderful texture you've been missing and make overly buttered toast seem soggy. You will even understand why the English serve toast in a rack to keep it dry and crisp instead of wrapping it up in a napkin as most American restaurants do, softening it and destroying the wonderful crunchiness of freshly toasted bread.

The only time it is actually necessary to give up food is when you decide to lose weight; then you must take in less fuel than you are burning. The extra fuel the body needs will then come from stored fuel or fat.

If, in the beginning, you are using *JET FUEL* primarily to lose fat, simply change the word *limit* to *avoid* so that you are not limiting your fat intake—you are *eliminating* it. You are not limiting the use of alcoholic beverages—you are *eliminating* them.

The word *diet* is not used in this book because it is obsolete. People who are into winning want to *gain* great bodies—not *lose* anything.

After following this program for only two or three days,

you are going to notice a marked difference in the way you feel, the amount of energy you have, and how much more clearly you think. After two weeks on *JET FUEL* everyone else is going to notice how fabulous you look and how much more positive your attitude has become about everything.

In the same two weeks you will save enough money following this program to more than pay for this book. Your food costs will continue to be at least one-third less than they have been. It is the only plan I know of in the present economy where less money gets you higher quality.

Your medical costs should also be greatly reduced because staying healthy often has far more to do with what you do for yourself than what the doctor does for you.

Remember—if you use the wrong kind of fuel in a jet engine and cause damage, you simply replace the damaged parts. *You* are issued only *one* body at birth, and it must last you for the rest of your life. Therefore, proper maintenance is essential for long-term performance.

IT'S IN TO BE FIT

Throughout history the lean look has come in and out of vogue. In England in the early nineteenth century, the ethereal, emaciated female body was considered attractive. Many women are said to have lived on a diet of vinegar and belladonna to achieve this almost sickly fragility.

It is no longer in just to be thin. It's in to be fit. Muscles have become the status symbol of fitness. Healthy is beautiful. Regular and adequate exercise has fortunately become such an important part of our culture that even party conversations now routinely include questions like "Where do you work out?" "How many laps do you swim?" or "What brand of running shoes do you wear?"

Exercise increases your metabolism.

Increased metabolism means that you are actually burning more calories every hour. This increase continues for a prolonged period of time after you have stopped exercising. When the metabolism is increased, stored energy is released, which keeps you from being as hungry. Exercise even helps control your appetite!

Because increased metabolism releases more stored fuel, it burns unwanted fat. The combination of *JET FUEL* and adequate exercise therefore burns fat, builds muscle, and keeps you *fit*.

Fitness includes strength, endurance, and flexibility. Your exercise program must be comprehensive to be effective.

Aerobic exercises are excellent for developing strength and endurance. Aerobic or cardiovascular activities exercise, work, and strengthen the heart muscle and allow for better oxygenation. Aerobic exercises include walking briskly, jogging, running, swimming, bicycling, jumping rope, or aerobic dancing—any exercise that keeps you in motion and elevates your heart rate.

You can become very strong and develop great endurance through aerobics and still not be flexible. Flexibility requires regular stretching exercises. Flexibility also contributes more to your body language than either strength or endurance. When watching someone walking at a distance, you can usually guess the person's age by the way he or she moves. We are often surprised to find that a person we judged from a distance to be hardly more than a teenager is in fact an agile senior citizen.

You can make exercise the central part of your life or you can build it into your current life-style with very little alteration. You can carry running shoes in your car and take every available opportunity to get out and go for a brisk walk. Get in the habit of stretching before and after you walk. There are some very good books available on aerobic exercises that can help you get started on a safe and rewarding program.

Regular exercise is necessary for good health and is certainly an integral part of the *JET FUEL* way of life. However, it is much easier to reduce body-fat levels by taking in less fuel than through exercising. The average person can burn 100 to 120 calories by running one mile. But the same person can avoid taking in the 100 to 120 calories in the first place by simply not eating the ice cream cone or buttering the bread.

This is the first time in our history that the fashionable look for both women and men has been linked to longevity and better health in general. The lean, fit look of the eighties is here to stay. No one is ever going to want to give up a look that goes with having more energy, a better sex life, and living longer. People on *JET FUEL* even smile a lot more!

The fact that you're looking better and feeling healthier and smarter brings with it the experience of *flying at full throttle*, perhaps for the first time in your life. It is a natural high—a new power dimension that continues to get better and better.

Although the press has tried to relate the fashionably fit look to an upper middle class phenomenon, there is really nothing elitist about it. The *JET FUEL* way of living is an attainable goal for people of all ages, races, and walks of life. All you need to do is decide to start *JET FUEL* living today.

Right now start visualizing yourself as stronger, smarter, and slimmer. Fit, successful people sit straighter, stand taller, and radiate a natural exuberance.

The great philosophers of the world have disagreed on many subjects; however they have all agreed on the most important force in life—that we become what we think we are. When you constantly visualize yourself as already looking and feeling fit and successful, you will reach that goal even more quickly.

Pretend you have a bunch of brightly colored helium-filled balloons attached to your sternum, the bone that holds your ribs together. The balloons constantly lift your chest up and out. Snap your belly button to your spine to flatten your stomach. Tighten your bottom and tuck it under for a nice straight back and beautiful posture. Now relax your knees as you walk forward—lifted by your balloons, stomach snapped in tightly—and smile. You will experience a marvelous sensation of floating and feel a wonderful new spring in your step.

With *JET FUEL* you are embarking on a flight pattern that *automatically* controls your nutritional intake *and* your weight. All you ever have to do is remember to apply the *JET FUEL* strategy of winning with food.

Whenever you are about to eat or drink anything remember your goals. Ask yourself:

"What do I want to look like?"

"How do I want to feel?"

"How do I want to perform?"

"Is my eating behavior helping me to achieve my goals?"

"Is it *JET FUEL?*"

JET FUEL is a positive force. It provides the energy for a dynamic life-style, good health, and an attitude of achievement.

Sit back, relax, and get ready to take off. You are going to learn everything you need to know about flying on *JET FUEL* in an hour. You are going to feel the incredible difference it is making in your life in less than a week.

Fuel Facts

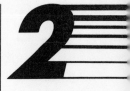

When taking off on *JET FUEL*, you'll need all of the basic information necessary for long-sustained flight, such as where calories come from, what the actual fuel sources are, and how additives can affect the quality of the fuel. Finally there are specific lists of preferred and limited fuel sources and additives for easy reference.

This information is especially important for men. Women are usually more informed about calorie sources and basic nutrition in general than men because women's magazines regularly include nutrition articles while men's publications rarely touch on the subject.

CALORIE DENSITY

You need to learn the meaning and the importance of calorie density so that you will never again have to count calories.

Calories come from only four sources: carbohydrates, protein, fat, and alcohol. Carbohydrates and protein contain four calories per gram. Fat contains nine calories per gram—over twice as many as either carbohydrates or protein. Alcohol contains seven calories per gram—almost twice as many as carbohydrates or protein. A gram is a unit of measurement in the metric system equal to .035 ounce; however, there is no need to convert to ounces because all ingredient labeling is given in grams.

Too many people have the wrong idea that cutting down on starchy foods such as breads, cereals, potatoes, and pastas and eating primarily protein food like fish, poultry, meat, eggs, and cheese are the best ways to cut calories. The fact is that a large percentage of these protein foods is fat, not protein. Since fat has more than twice as many calories as protein, instead of calorie cutting these people are actually calorie loading.

Picture yourself sitting at a table looking down at a plate with a steak, a baked potato, and a large serving of broccoli on it. The steak is the smallest item on the plate. The potato is half again bigger than the steak, and the broccoli is twice as big as the steak—yet they all weigh the same amount.

The potato and the broccoli contain more bulk and therefore weigh less for their volume than the steak.

Even though the steak is the smallest in size for its weight, it is the highest in calories. It has four times as many calories as the potato and almost twelve times as many calories as the broccoli.

You can certainly see that if you are trying to cut calories, the first thing to cut in half is the steak, not the potato, and certainly not the broccoli. If you are hungry and want more volume to eat without calorie loading—eat vegetables!

WATCH OUT FOR HIDDEN FAT

Potatoes are not fattening. It is the added fats that you put on baked potatoes, such as butter, margarine, sour cream, and chopped bacon, that are fattening because they are *fats*. Similarly it is not the protein in the steak that is fattening—it is the fat in the steak that is fattening! However, the difference is that you can leave the added fat off the baked potato but you can't get the fat out of the steak.

Here are several good examples of the dramatic calorie increase when fat is added:

- Two pats of butter spread on a whole wheat roll contain more calories than the roll itself.
- When eating pasta, think in terms of lots of pasta, lots less sauce. It's the sauce that contains the olive oil or butter and most of the calories.
- Just a few tablespoons of the average salad dressing contains more calories than the salad it is poured over.

Carbohydrates are the best fuel source for energy and burn faster than the fats. So not only are you taking in fewer calories, but you are burning up more calories, which gives you the energy to become stronger, smarter, and slimmer *faster*.

In general, vegetables offer the lowest calorie-density of all food groups. Fruits have a higher calorie-density than most vegetables and therefore cannot be totally unlimited. One piece of fruit with each meal and one as a snack is a recommended daily guideline. Dried fruits such as raisins, dates, prunes, and apricots have a higher calorie-density than fresh fruits because they are dehydrated. However, they are great for snacks because they can be carried with you so easily.

ALCOHOLIC BEVERAGES

Alcohol can give you an overload of calories. One or two drinks a day is the maximum for high-performance people who need the rest of their calorie intake to provide their vitamins, minerals, and fiber.

What is a drink? This is the next obvious question most people ask. A drink is one-half ounce of pure alcohol. Translated into usable terms, that is a jigger (one and a half ounces) of distilled spirits or hard liquor. It is also equivalent to two twelve-ounce glasses of beer or two five-ounce glasses of wine.

In other words, it is the alcohol that constitutes a drink rather than what you are drinking. I love it when I hear someone say, "I don't drink—I'll just have a glass of wine!" Alcohol is alcohol whether you are drinking a white wine spritzer or some tropical fruit juice and rum concoction decorated with a pineapple spear and a tiny paper parasol.

The calorie-density of alcoholic beverages can be spread out by adding more water or soda water for weaker mixed drinks, drinking Lite beer, and mixing wine with soda water for wine spritzers. Avoid liqueurs and sweet cocktails.

When drinking wine with a meal, always have a glass of water as well. Drinking the water alternately with the wine will help reduce the amount of wine you drink considerably. This way you don't have to give up the enjoyment of wine with your meal or live to regret drinking the next morning.

The calories of cocktails can be totally eliminated by drinking the Pilot's Cocktail. The Pilot's Cocktail is a delightfully refreshing nonalcoholic drink. It is aptly named for the person in control of the airplane. The pilot cannot drink alcoholic beverages either before or during flight. This offers an alternative that both looks like a drink and tastes like a drink. Directions for mixing the Pilot's Cocktail are on page 68.

LEARN TO TRADE OFF

The two single most important factors in calorie control are common sense and moderation. You want to be stronger, smarter, and slimmer—not feeling deprived. Trading off will help you accomplish your goals without ever having to give up anything you really want. Trading off simply means trading limited foods for each other. If you have butter or margarine on your toast for breakfast, use less salad dressing on your salad at lunch. If you want Roquefort dressing on your salad at lunch, use just enough for flavor—not enough to camouflage the taste of the other wonderful ingredients in the salad. And have fresh fruit for dessert—not cheesecake!

If you enjoy wine with your dinner, have a Pilot's Cocktail before dinner. If you prefer to have a drink before dinner, then forego the wine with the meal.

By learning to trade off properly, you'll never have to give up eating the food you like best. You can really have it all.

People who have junk-food hang-ups that they think they can't overcome always remind me of an episode on *The Mary Tyler Moore Show* when Rhoda was depressed and Mary kindly offered her some of the cottage cheese she was eating. Rhoda said, "Mary, cottage cheese doesn't solve anything. It's chocolate that solves everything."

The occasional junk-food freak-out never killed anyone —including Rhoda—or made anyone fat. It is one's total food and life-style strategy that is important.

FUEL SOURCES

CARBOHYDRATES (4 calories per gram)

Clean-burning "high-octane" fuel.

There are two categories of carbohydrates: *Simple carbohydrates* provide calories with no other nutritional benefit and are therefore a limited source of *JET FUEL*. Complex carbohydrates provide the best source of energy and are excellent sources of vitamins, minerals, and fiber. They are the most important source of *JET FUEL*.

Complex Carbohydrates

All of plant origin and all are unrefined. Includes fresh, natural fruits, vegetables, and grain products. Contains protein, sometimes fat. Contains fiber, which exists only in foods of plant origin. Contains *no* cholesterol, which is only found in foods of animal origin.

Dietary fiber is the indigestible part of plant food that cannot be absorbed by the body and does not supply calories. It absorbs moisture, adding bulk to the fuel mix, and speeds up the transit time of all other food through the body for proper bowel function. Because of this moisture absorption it is essential, on a high fiber diet, to drink an adequate amount of water. Many people think they cannot eat high fiber foods, simply because they don't drink enough water, and as a result experience painful stomachaches. The solution is to *drink* the necessary water.

Include all sugars and syrups. Refined flours and processed cereals are also best classified with the simple carbohydrates since most of their nutritional properties and fiber have been removed. Even when the labels say ENRICHED, not all of the nutrients are available and none of the fiber has been replaced.

Simple Carbohydrates

Sugars include any ingredient ending in *ose* such as sucrose, or ordinary table sugar; fructose; glucose; dextrose; lactose; maltose as well as corn syrup; maple syrup; honey; and molasses. Sugars provide calories but *no* nutrients of any significance—with the possible exception of blackstrap molasses, which has a high iron content. Honey has small quantities of minerals, but they are present in such infinitesimal amounts that they have no nutritional significance.

Sugars cause the blood sugar to rise rapidly, giving an immediate burst of energy, followed by a crash landing—a rapid drop in the blood sugar that causes feelings of hunger and weakness. This peak-and-valley effect is often referred to as sugar highs and lows. Also, *all* sugars contribute to tooth decay!

Sugars are hidden in many processed foods. For example, one tablespoon of catsup contains one teaspoon of sugar. Always read the labels.

Pure crystalline fructose is the sweetest of all sugars, so you can use less of it to attain the same level of sweetness, which offers a calorie advantage. It also does not result in the fall of blood sugar—the hungry feeling—which accompanies the intake of glucose, for fructose is not burned as rapidly and therefore does not have the same effect.

Sucrose (ordinary table sugar) is 50 percent glucose and 50 percent fructose. Honey varies, but is usually around 70 percent glucose and 30 percent fructose.

Don't confuse pure crystalline fructose with fructose corn syrups, which do contain glucose and do not offer the advantages of pure crystalline fructose. Foods high in ordinary table *sugar* include candy, cakes, pies, cookies, ice cream, soft drinks, and sweetened breakfast cereals.

You will be amazed at how much less frequently you dream about man-made sweets such as cakes and pies after getting used to sweet fresh fruit for dessert. Three medium bananas weighing over one pound have the same number of calories as two squares of chocolate, and are much more satisfying. The sugar contained in natural sources also provides a longer-lasting source of energy than man-made sweets, which are burned up rapidly.

Fruit is more filling because of the bulk and fiber it contains, and it satisfies the craving for something sweet rather than triggering a sweet binge. This is really important news for the "sweetaholic" or the "chocaholic."

FUEL SOURCES

The body's building blocks. Necessary for growth, maintenance, and repair of body cells.

    Contain essential minerals and amino acids. Slower-burning "lower octane" fuel than carbohydrates. Needed in combination with carbohydrates for long-sustained flight and good nutrition. *Available in foods of both plant and animal origin.*

PROTEINS (4 calories per gram)

Contains no fiber. Contains cholesterol.

    Cholesterol is a waxy substance found in all food of animal origin. It is also produced by the body. A certain amount of it is necessary for good health. However, when too much of it is present in the body, it can build up on the interior artery walls, narrowing and roughening the vessels through which blood must flow, causing atherosclerosis and heart disease. Egg yolks and animal fat have high cholesterol content, as do organ meats, some shellfish, caviar, and the skin of poultry. This does not mean that you can never eat eggs or other high cholesterol foods again, but it does mean you should practice the same trade-off policy that you do in controlling high fat foods.

    Animal protein also contains saturated fat, which is believed to contribute in the buildup of cholesterol.

Animal Protein

FUEL SOURCES

Fish, Poultry, and Meat

Fish is lower in fat than poultry or meat and the best source of animal protein.

Chicken, when eaten without skin, is lower in fat than most meat.

Meat is divided into three grades: prime, choice, and good. The grades are determined by how well marbled the meat is. Marbling consists of streaks of fat running through the red muscle of the meat. Good contains the least amount of fat. Avoid prime cuts of meat. Limit red meat to three servings a week.

Dairy Products

Divided into categories depending on the amount of butterfat they contain.

Milk

1 Cup (8 ounces)	Butterfat Content
Nonfat (skim) milk	No butterfat
Low-fat (2 percent) milk	1 pat (1 teaspoon) butter
Whole milk	2 pats (2 teaspoons) butter

Remember—the next time you want a glass of whole milk, you are actually reaching for one glass of nonfat milk *and* two pats of butter.

Look for label indicating reduced fat content such as nonfat or low-fat yogurt, low-fat cottage cheese, part-skim ricotta, or part-skim mozzarella.	**Other Dairy Products**

Contains fiber. Contains no cholesterol.
    Legumes are the richest sources of vegetable protein. They include all dried peas and beans, peanuts, and soybeans. Foods made from soybeans such as tofu, which is soybean curd, are also good substitutes for animal protein.
    The protein quality of legumes is improved by combining them with rice, corn, or grains.
    Nuts and seeds are also good sources of vegetable protein; however, they contain too much fat to be used as a regular source of vegetable protein when mixing *JET FUEL*. Use them only occasionally for flavor and texture.
	Vegetable Protein

The body's natural enemy. Leading source of calories with little nutritional benefit. Fat builds up on your stomach, hips and thighs, and even around your neck to make you look older and less attractive. It builds up inside the blood vessels and around the organs and interferes with	**FAT (9 calories per gram)**

good health. It even makes it more difficult to move around. It is not necessary to add any fat in a well-balanced eating program. Enough fat is available in animal protein and complex carbohydrates without adding extra fat.

There are three types of fats:

Saturated fats are all fats of animal origin as well as coconut and palm oils. These contribute to the buildup of cholesterol in the blood vessels.

Polyunsaturated fats include vegetable oils such as safflower and corn oil. These aid in reducing the cholesterol buildup in the blood vessels. Polyunsaturated fats are liquid at room temperature; the softer the polyunsaturated fat source, the higher the percentage of polyunsaturated fat. Therefore, tub margarine is a better source of polyunsaturated fat than stick margarine.

Monounsaturated fats contribute neither to the buildup nor to the breakdown of cholesterol —they just add calories. These include nuts, nut oils, avocados, olives, and olive oil.

Since all fats have the same nine calories in every gram, it is best to select fats in the polyunsaturated category when adding them for flavor or moisture.

Alcohol, like fat and sugar, has no nutritional value except adding calories. These three fuel sources are often called empty calories because they contain no vitamins, minerals, or fiber. Therefore if you want to lose weight or maintain that lean, fit look, it is important to use moderation when drinking any alcoholic beverages. Limit your intake to one or two drinks a day. This includes beer and wine as well as distilled alcohol such as vodka, gin, rum, Scotch, and bourbon.

ALCOHOL (7 calories per gram)

The "double trouble" of alcohol is that it lowers the blood sugar, causing you to become hungry, *and* it goes directly to the judgment center of the brain, lowering your willpower at the same time. This combination of increased appetite and decreased willpower will cause you to eat ordinary fuel that you normally wouldn't eat *and* to take in more fuel than you need.

WATER

Just as a turbojet is a glutton for air, the body should be a glutton for water. *It will not rust you!*

Adequate water is necessary to dilute the impurities or waste materials constantly being excreted by the body so that the kidneys are not overworked. Six to eight glasses of plain water a day will not only improve your general health; it will give you beautiful clear skin. Water also acts as a natural diuretic. It's just like priming a pump —the more water you drink, the less you retain. Water also helps prevent overheating and dehydration.

Coffee, tea, and diet drinks are *not* water substitutes! Six to eight glasses of water mean just that—six to eight glasses of pure water. In fact, both coffee and alcohol speed up dehydration.

Bottled water is best and is especially important in those areas of the country where the sodium content of the drinking water is high. Distilled water contains no sodium.

Naturally occurring sparkling waters such as Perrier, Poland, Calistoga, and low-sodium soda waters are lower in sodium than regular soda water.

SALT (sodium)

Salt is sodium chloride. *Salt is not a food and does not contain calories.* If you eat too much sodium, fluid accumulates in the body, causing you to look and feel bloated. Many people falsely believe salt is fattening because the fluid retention increases weight on the scale. It is also dangerous because the increased blood volume makes the heart work harder and causes blood pressure to rise, a condition called hypertension.

One level teaspoon of salt contains 1,938 milligrams of sodium. According to the American Heart Association, no one needs more than 2000 milligrams a day. Sodium is present in varying degrees in *all* foods, so always taste food before adding salt. Foods high in sodium include most cheeses, many condiments, canned soups and sauces, celery, sauerkraut, pickles, and olives.

After you consciously reduce the amount of salt you use in cooking and avoid adding salt to your meals whenever possible, you will find that you almost immediately lose your taste for salty foods—even if you were a salt addict who salted first, then tasted.

If your store does not carry low-sodium products, write to The Low Sodium Pantry, 4901 Auburn Avenue, Bethesda, Maryland 20814 for a catalog describing the most complete line.

Salt Substitutes

They are made from potassium and have a terrible metallic aftertaste when heated. Some substitutes also contain sodium and should be used sparingly.

ARTIFICIAL SWEETENERS

Artificial sweeteners are not good substitutes because they contain chemicals that the body does not need to function properly, and some are potentially dangerous. Also, they distort the perception of natural sweetness. It is better to use a small amount of sugar, which contains only sixteen calories a teaspoon. Foods high in artificial sweeteners include most so-called diet desserts and diet soft drinks.

Ironically none of the sugar substitutes has ever been shown to help weight loss. In fact, it is doubtful that they make any difference in tooth decay because most common decay-promoting foods are not sweetened with sugar substitutes.

CAFFEINE

Caffeine is a drug that stimulates the adrenal glands to produce more adrenaline, which then acts as a stimulant, giving you a false sense of energy. Caffeine actually lowers the blood sugar, giving you a low that is hidden by the high you feel as long as the adrenaline is keeping you stimulated. As soon as the adrenaline wears off, you have less energy because of lowered blood sugar, and you also feel hungry. If you continue this cycle of drinking more coffee or tea for more energy, you will get what is often called coffee nerves, a shaky, irritable feeling.

Caffeine has other side effects such as sleeplessness, anxiety, gastritis, and heartburn, and has recently been associated with the growth of fibrous cysts in women's breasts. Caffeine is found in coffee, tea, chocolate, cola beverages, and many soft drinks.

Decaffeinated Coffee

Decaffeinated coffee contains less than six milligrams of caffeine per five-ounce cup, compared to regular coffee, which has about ninety milligrams of caffeine per five-ounce cup. Therefore, if you drink too much decaffeinated coffee, it will have the same effect on you as drinking regular coffee.

Some decaffeinated coffee is still decaffeinated by a chemical process that has been shown to cause cancer in laboratory animals. Make sure any decaffeinated coffee you drink has been decaffeinated by the Swiss, or water-washed, method.

Complex Carbohydrates

Whole-grain products
  Breads and rolls
  Tortillas
  Grains and cereals—Barley, brown rice, buckwheat groats (kasha), corn meal, popcorn, cracked wheat (bulgur), millet, old-fashioned oatmeal, multigrain cereals, and rye
  Cold cereals—Puffed rice, corn, and wheat; shredded wheat; Grape-Nuts; and *JET FUEL!*

Vegetables

Legumes—Richest source of vegetable protein. Includes all dried peas and beans, such as lentils, black-eyed peas, chick-peas (garbanzo beans), kidney beans, navy beans, pinto beans, black beans, peanuts, soybeans, and foods made from soybeans.

Tofu—Soybean curd. Excellent source of vegetable protein.

Fruits and dried fruits

Animal Protein

Fish

Poultry

Meat—Buy good *not* choice or prime grades.

Dairy products
  Nonfat milk
  Buttermilk—Higher in sodium than other milks, but calories are usually the same as nonfat or low-fat milk.
  Nonfat dry milk powder—Available in two forms, instant and noninstant. Instant can be mixed in water with a spoon. Noninstant must be mixed in a blender. When you need milk, just mix the dry powder and water.
  Skimmed evaporated canned milk—Twice the calories per cup of nonfat milk because it is condensed.
  Nonfat and low-fat yogurt—Avoid fruit-flavored yogurts because they contain sugar.
  Low-fat cheeses:
    Cottage cheese—Low-fat only
    Ricotta and mozzarella—Partially skimmed (also sold as part-skim)
    Romano and Parmesan—Use sparingly; high in sodium

Canned Goods

Vegetables—When fresh are not available; tomato products such as tomato sauce, purée, and paste, all of which are excellent bases for sauces. Also available with no salt added.

Fruits—Packed in water or natural juice only. No sugar added.

PREFERRED FUEL

Fish—Tuna and other canned seafood, water-packed. Also available with no salt added.

Stock (chicken or beef), often called broth—Preferable to powdered or bouillon cubes; closer to the flavor of homemade stock and contains less salt. Also available with no salt added.

Juices
Fruit—Unsweetened only; when fresh fruit juices are not available.
Tomato and vegetable—Available with no salt added.

Frozen Foods

Juices and fruits—Unsweetened; when fresh fruit juices are not available.

Vegetables—Unsalted; when fresh vegetables are not available.

Seasonings and Condiments

Herbs and spices,* both dried and fresh—When possible, purchase dried herbs and spices in jars with tight-fitting lids to preserve freshness. To buy all of the herbs and spices you will want at one time would destroy your budget. I recommend your own Spice-of-the-Week

* Calorie-free

Club, adding the herb or spice you need each week for a new recipe or trying the suggested uses you will find on the labels.

Extracts*—There are many others besides vanilla, so buy one a week and experiment, expecially with desserts. Try coconut, rum, almond, and mint extracts to start.

Vinegars*—Many varieties; needed for salad dressings, sauces, and marinades

Tabasco*—Taste between drops—very hot!

Mustard—Experiment with different varieties, such as Dijon, spicy brown, and horseradish. Lower in fat and sugar than most condiments. Available in low sodium if necessary.

Liquid smoke products*—Good flavor for barbecue sauce or any other dish in which you want a smoky flavor.

Worcestershire sauce*—Use sparingly; high in sodium.

Soy sauce*—Use sparingly; high in sodium. Try reduced-sodium variety.

Pickles—Use sparingly; high in sodium.

* Calorie-free

PREFERRED FUEL

Water	Drinking water, distilled water, and sparkling water
Herb Tea	Caffeine-free; the most popular herb teas are orange, mint, cinnamon, and chamomile. A caffeine-free product must be labeled CAFFEINE-FREE.

Simple Carbohydrates

Sugar and syrups

Refined grain products
   White flour
   White bread and rolls
   Highly processed cereals and cereals contain-
      ing sugar
   Candy, cookies, cakes, and pies

Animal Protein

Meat—choice and prime grades

High-fat dairy products
   Whole milk
   Low-fat milk
   Whole yogurt
   Half-and-half
   Cream
   Butter—High in saturated fat and cholesterol;
      pure corn oil or safflower oil margarines are
      good polyunsaturated, cholesterol-free sub-
      stitutes, but have the same number of fat
      calories.
   Sour cream
   Ice cream—High in fat
   Ice milk—Lower in fat than ice cream
   High-fat cheeses—Also high in sodium.
      Cheddar, Jack, Swiss, Roquefort, Camem-
      bert, Brie, Bleu, Edam, Liederkranz,
      Muenster, pimiento and other spreads.

Eggs—Egg yolks are high in cholesterol.

Vegetable Protein	Nuts and seeds—High in fat; always buy raw nuts and seeds with the exception of peanuts. Buy dry-roasted, unsalted peanuts. Peanut butter—High in fat; always buy unhomogenized.
Fats	Margarine—High in polyunsaturated fat. Contains no cholesterol (same calories as butter); use only pure corn oil or pure safflower oil margarine. Read the labels—some less expensive margarines contain coconut or palm oil, which are saturated fats. Tub margarine is better than stick margarine. Oil—High in fat; use corn or safflower oil or other polyunsaturated oil. Read the labels— avoid coconut and palm oils, which are saturated fats. Coconut and palm oils are also found in many nondairy cream and milk substitutes and some margarines. Mayonnaise—High in fat
Beverages	Coffee—Contains caffeine Decaffeinated coffee—Contains smaller amounts of caffeine; make sure any decaffeinated coffee you drink has been decaffeinated by the Swiss, or water-washed, method.

Tea—Contains caffeine

Cocoa—Contains caffeine

Soft drinks—Contain sugar and often contain caffeine

Diet sodas—Contain artificial sweeteners and often contain caffeine

Wine, beer, and liquor—High in calories and offer little nutritional value; however, acceptable for cooking. Adds flavor, and the alcohol evaporates in the cooking process.

Miscellaneous Canned goods—Avoid all products with added salt, sugar, or preservatives.

Frozen foods—Avoid all products with added salt, sugar, or preservatives.

Catsup—High in sodium and sugar

Olives—High in fat and sodium

Salt

Salt substitutes

Artificial sweeteners—Contain chemical additives

Modern Marketing and Streamlining the Galley

3

Now that you know what you need to mix *JET FUEL,* the next step is to modernize your marketing and storing methods to make food preparation faster, more efficient, and less expensive. The buying, storing, and preparation of food should be well-organized, easy, and even fun.

The first step to shopping is the list. Keep the list on the wall of your kitchen all the time. Each time you run low on anything, write it on the list. Never wait until you are out of it. Then, before going to the market, plan your weekly menu and add all of the ingredients necessary to your shopping list.

Always include emergency supplies for unexpected occasions. If you are planning to entertain during the week, everything you need for your party should also be included on your list. Items such as cocktail napkins and candles can often be purchased in a supermarket and save you the time and trouble of making a special trip for them later in the week. You may find the sample shopping list on page 41 helpful in organizing your own shopping list.

When possible, plan to shop only once a week. Schedule your shopping trip just as you would schedule any other appointment. Don't minimize the importance of food—make it a part of your routine. Shopping time should include the time necessary to write your shopping list, actually do the shopping, and store your groceries properly when you return.

Writing your shopping list according to the geographical layout of your market is important for the best use of your time. Practically all supermarkets are designed the same way. You will find most of the *JET FUEL* on the walls. On one wall are the fresh fruits and vegetables. On another wall you will find fresh fish, poultry, and meat. The dairy products and basic bread items are also on the walls. What does that leave in the middle aisles? The ordinary and the inferior fuels! There are obvious exceptions to this rule, such as grains, cereals, herbs and spices, some frozen and canned goods, and of course, cleaning products, paper supplies, and drug items. The shopping list you take with you should list all of the items you need in the middle aisles by category so that they are easy to find.

Just as soon as you have everything on your list that's in the middle of the market, run for the walls. Don't allow yourself the time to be manipulated by the clever advertisers trying to turn you into a shopping robot. There are thousands of different food products loaded with fat, sugar, and salt cleverly concealed by misleading labeling. Be aware of popular gimmicks in labeling such as VITAMIN AND MINERAL FORTIFIED. The misleading information can make even real junk food appear to be *JET FUEL*. Ingredients must be listed in order of amounts by weight. When you see a breakfast cereal with the first ingredient listed as *sugar,* you can be certain that it is not *JET FUEL*.

There are certain limited fuels which are especially tempting to everyone. They are different for different people. For example, ice cream may be one person's weakness and

SHOPPING LIST

MIDDLE AISLES

Cereals, Grains, Pasta,
Dried Beans, Flour,
Baking Needs

Canned Goods

Frozen Foods

Condiments, Herbs,
Spices, Extracts

Beverages: Bottled
Water, Etc.

Cleaning Products
and Paper Supplies

Drug Items

WALLS

Vegetables

Fruit

Dairy, Eggs

Fish, Poultry, Meat

Breads

Other Stores

high-fat cheese such as Camembert or Brie another's. Salty nuts and potato chips have their addicts as well. Buying and storing the limited fuels that are most tempting to you is courting disaster. Restrain yourself while shopping—it will make it so much easier for you at home.

One-stop shopping may not always be possible. It may be necessary to go to a health food store for some of the items you need, such as raw nuts and seeds, and some whole grain products or to a fish market for fresh fish and seafood. You may even have a favorite produce market or bakery in which you can shop conveniently more frequently than once a week.

When planning your weekly menu, allow leeway in selection of fresh fruits and vegetables. Choose some of the fresh produce at the market, selecting the best quality available. In-season fruits and vegetables are always the best buy. They look better, have more flavor, and are less expensive. When buying meat, be aware of the three main grades: prime, choice, and good. Remember—good contains the least amount of fat and is by far the best source of *JET FUEL* in the meat category. It is also the least expensive!

Schedule your shopping at a time when you are not hungry. If the only time available is at the end of the day, have a *JET FUEL* snack to take the edge off your appetite before marketing. A banana is ideal because it grows its own wrapper—just peel and eat! Also if you are coming right from the office, have a pair of comfortable shoes in your car to change into. Running shoes are in.

When planning time in your weekly schedule for shopping, always include enough time to wash and store all of your vegetables properly. This not only saves time later when you are going to use them; it also adds greatly to their life spans and saves money because there is much less spoilage.

All leafy vegetables such as lettuce, spinach, and parsley should be torn apart completely and soaked in cold water until completely free of all dirt. Drain the leaves thoroughly and then roll them in towels or put them in bags before refrigerating them. When you are ready to prepare a salad, your lettuce is clean, crisp, and *dry*. Dryness is very important. Wet lettuce dilutes the salad dressing so that you need more of it. Most salad dressings add enormously to the calorie-density of each serving.

Root vegetables such as carrots, parsnips, turnips, beets, and potatoes should be washed and dried before storing in the refrigerator, but don't peel or scrape them until you are ready to use them.

Fruit should also be washed and dried but not peeled or cut until you are ready to use it. If the fruit is ripe, put it in the refrigerator to slow down further ripening. If it is not completely ripe, leave it out at room temperature until it is ripe and then refrigerate until you are ready to use it. Bananas are the exception. They will turn brown if refrigerated. If bananas are getting too ripe, peel and slice them and store in plastic bags in the freezer to use later for milk shakes, cereal toppings, or banana bread.

Whenever I hear people say, "Oh, I couldn't possibly take the time to wash and dry my vegetables before storing them," I ask them, "Do you eat dirty salads?" The truth is that you will choose to eat *JET FUEL* more frequently when it is already clean and ready to eat than if you have to stop to wash and dry it first.

After packages of dried fruits are opened, they should also be stored in the refrigerator in covered containers to prevent further dehydration, keeping them fresh and soft longer.

Jet Age bugs are smarter than many Jet Age people— they already prefer whole-grain products to their boring refined counterparts. This includes breads, cereals, pastas, and flour. Even if you seal the whole-grain flours and cereals in airtight containers in the cupboards, the bugs manage to get to them. Then you have the problem of getting rid of the bugs. This means throwing away all of your bug-infested inventory, including many dry herbs, because when the bugs get in, they take over. This discarding and replacing is both time-consuming *and* expensive.

Refrigerating these natural products will also ensure their freshness and full flavor for a longer period of time. The oils in many whole grains, nuts, and seeds will turn rancid quickly when not refrigerated.

If you do not use much bread, it is best to keep it in the freezer to be used as needed. Either thaw it to room temperature or put the frozen bread in the toaster to eat immediately. Pastas, rice, and cooked cereals can be prepared in larger quantities than needed and then frozen in serving sizes for future meals.

Canned stock or broth should be kept in the refrigerator so that the fat congeals on the top and can be removed easily after opening.

Other items which should be refrigerated after opening either to retain their flavor or to prevent spoilage include coffee (decaffeinated by the water method), pickles, peanut butter, mustard, and mayonnaise.

Tofu (soybean curd) should be refrigerated. After opening the package, place any remaining tofu in fresh water or in juice or stock if you wish to add flavor.

When storing anything in either the refrigerator or the freezer, it is important to cover it tightly so that the air cannot get to it. This prevents dehydration, which causes loss of taste and texture. Also, unless dairy products are tightly covered in the refrigerator, they will pick up the taste of other foods.

With fuel supplies organized, you are ready to turn your attention to streamlining your kitchen for easy access, maximum efficiency, and minimum preparation time.

Keep adequate supplies for proper storage, such as plastic bags, plastic wrap, aluminum foil, plastic containers, and jars with tight-fitting lids.

Arrange your herbs and spices in a cool place where they are never exposed to sunlight and alphabetize them for easy access. This may not seem important to you now, but as you acquire more herbs and spices it will save you time *and* frustration.

Extracts such as almond, coconut, mint, rum, and vanilla are also easier to find in a hurry if you have them in alphabetical order.

The most important work simplification rule is to have the things you are using within reach when you need them. Organize your equipment so that the items you use most and the foods you eat most often are the most accessible. When possible, free up as much counter space as you can so that you have adequate work area for meal preparation.

JET FUEL is not only cleaner-burning fuel; it also makes cooking cleaner *and* cleanup easier! Since you use little or no butter, margarine, or oil in *JET FUEL* preparation, there is no grease on your stove, and there are no greasy pans to wash. Grease just adds work, wastes time—and makes you fat!

JET FUEL
in Transition
From Raw Materials to Menus

You are going to learn all the tricks necessary for turning *JET FUEL* out of your galley easily. You will also be surprised at how fast *JET FUEL* can be prepared.

Cooking the *JET FUEL* way, you will be using much less fat without anyone noticing the difference, using less sugar without giving up sweets, and adding much less salt without ever missing it.

You will also happily discover how much you really like vegetables when they are cooked properly. You will learn how to combine vegetables with grain products for entrées that greatly cut your food costs while adding interest and variety to your menus.

Before going into the kitchen you should be in the proper uniform. Always work in tight-fitting clothes. Tight jeans are ideal. If you wear flowing caftans or big shirts and baggy pants, you will eventually grow to fit them. Tight clothes make you much more aware of your body. You stand up straighter and more easily avoid the kitchen malady I call hand-to-mouth disease—or tasting while you're cooking. This "tasting" often amounts to more fuel intake than the average meal!

REDUCING THE AMOUNT OF FAT

Avoid frying or sautéing in oil, butter, or margarine

Cook in nonstick cookware or use nonstick spray in other cookware. When using nonstick cookware, cook over very low heat. You can cook fish, poultry, meat, eggs, or pancakes in this manner.

Use water, defatted stock, juice, or wine instead of butter, margarine, or oil to prevent sticking and burning.

Start with the onions! Put chopped or sliced onions in a pan with a lid. Cook, covered, over very low heat, stirring occasionally until the onions are tender and clear. If they are cooked slowly enough, the onions release their own moisture and do not need any fat or additional liquid to prevent sticking or burning. To the onions you can then add fish, poultry, meat, or any vegetable. Cover and cook until done. When you use this method, the onions impart such wonderful flavor to anything you are cooking that no extra seasoning is needed.

Bake, broil, poach, or steam

When baking fish, poultry, or meat, you can save time by avoiding dirty baking dishes. Wrap what you are cooking in aluminum foil like an envelope. Add any herbs, spices, stock, juice, or wine you are using before sealing the end of the envelope.

After baking, use the liquid in the envelope

to pour over vegetables. It is a delicious, almost calorie-free sauce.

Fat-free stock

It is best to make your own stock if you have the time. Use any stock recipe, omitting or reducing the salt. Strain the stock and then refrigerate it until it is cold and the fat congeals on the top. Remove the fat and place the stock in the freezer in the size containers you will need. You can freeze it in ice-cube trays and then place the cubes in plastic bags; the cubes may be used 1 or 2 at a time for sautéing or for adding flavor to sauces.

The advantage of making your own stock is that it tastes better, has a lower sodium content, *and* is much less expensive.

If you don't want to bother making your own, then buy canned stock or broth, but remember—keeping it in the refrigerator makes it easy to remove the fat when you open the can.

Bouillon cubes and powdered stocks are so salty that they are not good substitutes and should be used only in emergencies.

Fat-free soups

Defatted stock and consommé are easy, almost calorie-free soups. Add a little sherry for sherried consommé or turn your defatted stock into egg drop soup by bringing it to a boil and whipping an egg into it. For lower-cholesterol egg drop soup, use only the egg whites. Add low-sodium soy sauce to taste and garnish with chopped green onion tops.

Fat-free drippings

Remove fat from pan drippings by pouring them into a bowl and placing the bowl in the refrigerator until all of the fat has solidified at the top. Remove the fat for fat-free drippings. Faster method: Place the bowl in the freezer. After 20 minutes you can remove the fat. Fat-free drippings can be kept in the freezer to be added to stock for extra flavor and to make fat-free gravy.

Fat-free gravy

You can make fat-free gravy by combining 1 tablespoon of cornstarch or arrowroot with 2 tablespoons cold water and adding the paste to a cup of defatted pan drippings. Simmer until thickened and season as desired.

Fat-free sauces

Use fat-free stock or fat-free drippings as the base of your sauces. You can also boil wine in a saucepan, reducing it in volume by one-third. Then combine it with a fat-free stock and thicken it with a little cornstarch dissolved in cold water. This makes a wonderful low-calorie imitation of a classic brown sauce. To get the rich dark color associated with the classic French brown sauce, add a little Kitchen Bouquet.

Fat-free barbecue sauce

Combine canned tomato sauce with a few drops of a liquid smoke product.

Low-fat sauces

Use less butter, margarine, or oil than called for in your recipe. Use nonfat milk instead of whole milk or cream. Making white sauce with nonfat milk takes longer for it to thicken.

Fat-free and low-fat salad dressings

It is always better to make your own salad dressings. It will be better in flavor, contain no preservatives, and be much less expensive. Classic salad dressings have a ratio of 2 parts oil to 1 part vinegar. A fraction of this amount of oil is necessary to make the dressing cling to the greens. Use your own favorite dressing recipe, using only a few tablespoons of oil instead of a cup or two. Or completely eliminate the oil with *JET FUEL* Dressing. It is a simple, tasty dressing that can be made in minutes in a jar with a tight-fitting lid. Combine ½ cup red wine vinegar, ¼ teaspoon freshly ground black pepper, ½ teaspoon salt, 1 tablespoon fructose, 2 garlic cloves, minced (or ½ teaspoon garlic powder), 2 teaspoons Worcestershire sauce, 1 tablespoon Dijon mustard, and the juice of ½ lemon. Screw the lid on tightly and shake well. Add ½ cup water and again shake well. Store in the refrigerator. If you want to vary the seasoning, add one of the following: for tarragon dressing, 1 tablespoon tarragon; for Italian dressing, a combination of 1 teaspoon each of tarragon, oregano, and basil; for Mexican dressing, ½ teaspoon ground cumin; and for Oriental dressing, 1 teaspoon curry powder. If you want a little heavier dressing, add 3 or 4 tablespoons of corn oil or safflower oil before adding the water. If you want a creamy dressing, add a little low-fat yogurt or cottage cheese and mix thoroughly. Start using your imagination and create your own "house dressing." It is even fun to bottle it for gifts. Once you get used to less oil in your dressing, ordinary salad dressings will taste greasy.

Low-fat dips

Use nonfat or low-fat yogurt or low-fat cottage cheese to replace sour cream in your own favorite recipes. Try combining equal parts of yogurt and cottage cheese in the blender and blend until completely smooth. Then season as you would a sour cream dip.

Low-fat dips also make wonderful spreads for bread and crackers. Try using them instead of butter on your toast for breakfast.

Nonfat "cream" | Combine nonfat dry milk with much less water than is necessary to make milk for a thicker, creamier mixture.

Nonfat whipped "cream" | You can make a whipped cream–type topping with nonfat dry milk. Chill the bowl and beater. Combine ⅓ cup nonfat dry milk and ⅓ cup ice water in the chilled bowl. Beat 3 to 4 minutes on high speed until soft peaks form. Add 2 tablespoons fresh lemon juice and beat 3 to 4 minutes longer, until stiff. Makes about 3½ cups.

You can also make whipped "cream" with canned skimmed evaporated milk. Chill it until it is very cold. Chill the bowl and beater. Whip it until it expands to five times its volume. Use immediately because it will quickly return to its liquid state. However, it can be chilled and whipped again.

Nonfat jelled milk | Soften an envelope of gelatin in 2 tablespoons cool water. Add 3 tablespoons of boiling water and stir until gelatin is completely dissolved. Then add 2 cups nonfat milk, mix well, cover, and store in the refrigerator until jelled.

Jelled milk makes a wonderful creamy sauce or topping. Just put the jelled milk in a blender and flavor as desired. Blend until smooth and then pour over fruit or cereal.

For a milk pudding, pour it into bowls or sherbet glasses and let it stand in the refrigerator until it has rejelled.

Eggs Hard-boiled egg whites can be used for garnishing soups, salads, and other dishes. Beaten raw egg whites substitute surprisingly well for whole eggs in many recipes. Even scrambled eggs and omelets can be made with one egg yolk and two or three whites.

REDUCING THE AMOUNT OF SUGAR

You can raise the level of perceived sweetness without adding any sweetener by using vanilla extract and/or cinnamon. You can often substitute concentrated fruit juice (frozen undiluted orange, apple, or pineapple) for the sweetener in recipes calling for sugar. You can almost always reduce the amount of sugar called for in a recipe by at least one-third and usually one-half. You can always reduce it by at least one-third if you use fructose instead of sucrose (ordinary table sugar) because it is one and one-half times sweeter. (Fructose is available in most supermarkets and in all health food stores.) Fructose can be substituted in all recipes except those for candy, because it does not make candy harden

properly. This fact should be of little conse-
quence to people flying on *JET FUEL,* since you
are not likely to be making candy!

REDUCING THE AMOUNT OF SALT

Remember—we taste only sweet, salt, sour, and
bitter. Everything else is smell. Salt is used to
heighten or sharpen flavors, so when using less
salt, it is necessary to add more "smell." The
same level of taste can be achieved by using up
to two to three times as many herbs and spices.
Stock, juices, and/or wine can replace water for
added flavor. Stimulating the other taste buds
with something sweet, sour, or bitter such as
fructose or concentrated fruit juice, fresh lemon
juice, or vinegar are also helpful in keeping you
from missing the salt.

You will find that after you have started
consciously reducing the amount of added salt
in your food, you actually lose your taste for it.
Canned soups and the soups served in most restaurants will taste like they have been made with
salt water!

I call salt the great dietary whitewash. If
something doesn't taste quite right—add salt!
Actually if it is seasoned just right, you don't
need the salt!

USING HERBS AND SPICES

Herbs and spices contain no calories and add greatly to the flavor and enjoyment of food.

When using dried herbs and spices that are not powdered, it is essential to crush them, using a mortar and pestle, before adding them to recipes. This releases their full aroma for maximum flavor. You will be amazed at how much better everything tastes. Salad dressings, sauces, and casseroles will have a fuller, more satisfying flavor with appreciably less or *no* salt added. Everyone will think you are a much improved cook.

There are a number of good herb mixtures now on the market that are completely free of salt and that provide interesting flavors for all types of dishes. Look for them in your grocery store.

It is also fun to grow your own herbs. Fresh herbs enhance the flavor of any food and make unusual and attractive garnishes on your plate.

It is the seasoning that adds the character to dishes of all types. You can change the whole personality of a recipe by changing only the herbs and spices. For example, you could take a basic chicken recipe and change the flavor to Italian by adding oregano; to French by adding tarragon; to Spanish by adding a little saffron; to Oriental by adding a little curry powder and ginger; and to Mexican by adding ground cumin and chili powder.

USING VEGETABLES

Steaming vegetables is the best method of cooking them. All you need is a collapsible steamer basket and a pot with a lid to put it in. You place enough water in the pot to bring it to a point just below the steam-basket level. Bring the water to a boil and put the vegetables in the steamer basket into the pot. Cover and set your timer, using the steaming chart on pages 58-59 as a guide.

As soon as the vegetables are cooked, remove the steamer basket from the pot and place it under cold running water. This preserves both the color and the texture of the vegetables. At this point you may wish to refrigerate your steamed vegetables and serve them cold or reheat them later to be served hot.

This is the way vegetables are prepared in many restaurants, which is why their vegetables are always so crisp and brightly colored. They can be reheated easily in a little defatted chicken broth or sautéed in butter, adding herbs and spices of your choice. Also, having cold cooked vegetables on hand in the refrigerator gives you the basis of marinated salads, imaginative soups, entrées—and great snacks.

People have told me that they do not like cooking cabbage, cauliflower, or broccoli because of the odor that permeates the house. If you can smell vegetables cooking, you have overcooked them! The problem of odor in the house from vegetables should be over for you forever, simply by using the steaming chart.

══ VEGETABLE STEAMING CHART ══

Vegetable	Minutes	Vegetable	Minutes
Artichokes*	30–45	Chicory	1–2
Asparagus	5	Chives	2–3
Beans:		Collards	1–2
butter	5	Corn	3
green	5	Coriander (cilantro)	1–2
hyacinth	5	Cucumber**	2
lima	5	Dandelion greens	1–2
string or snap	5	Eggplant**	5
wax	5	Endive	1–2
Bean sprouts	1–2	Escarole	1–2
Beet greens	3–5	Garlic	5
Beets**	15	Goboroot (black root)**	5
Black-eyed peas	5	Jerusalem artichokes	8
Black radish**	5	Jicama**	5
Breadfruit**	10	Kale	1–2
Broccoli:		Kohlrabi**	8–10
florets	3–5	Leeks**	5
branches	5	Lettuce	1–2
Brussels sprouts	5	Lotus root**	25
Cabbage, quartered:	5	Mushrooms	2
Chinese	3	Mustard, fresh	1–2
Carrots**	5	Okra	5
Cauliflower:		Onions:**	5
florets	3	green tops (scallions)	3
whole	5	pearl onions	5
Celery root**	3–4	Palm hearts	5
Celery ribs	10	Parsley	1–2
Chard	1–2	Parsnips**	15
Chayote**	3	Pea pods	3

VEGETABLE STEAMING CHART

Vegetable	Minutes	Vegetable	Minutes
Peas	3–5	Rutabagas**	8
Peppers:		Shallots	2
chili	2–3	Sorrel (dock)	2
bell**	2	Spinach	1–2
Pimientos	2	Squash:**	
Pokeweed	3	acorn or Hubbard	5
Potatoes:**		summer or zucchini	3
sweet	15	Tomatoes	3
white	10	Turnips**	8
Pumpkin**	5	Turnip greens	2
Radishes	5	Water chestnuts	8
Rhubarb	5	Watercress	1–2
Romaine lettuce	1–2		

* When steaming artichokes, do not use a steamer basket. Place them, heart side down, in just enough water to cover the heart area. Add fresh sliced lemon to the water. Bring the water to a boil, cover, and steam 30 to 45 minutes or until a leaf can be pulled easily from the heart. Steaming time depends on the size of the artichoke.

** Cut into ½" slices

Cooked vegetables can be the bases for fast, delicious meals such as vegetables au gratin. Put them in a baking or au gratin dish, sprinkle grated cheese over the top, and heat them until the vegetables are hot and the cheese is melted.

For a really simple vegetable casserole, cook onions until soft and clear and combine them with chopped steamed vegetables in a baking dish. Use approximately one onion and two cups of the steamed vegetables for each person. Sprinkle grated cheese over the top and place in a preheated 350° oven until the mixture is just heated through and the cheese is melted. You don't even need any additional seasoning.

I call my own favorite vegetable combination Broccoli à la Häringe for the famous castle just outside Stockholm where I first made it. Add sliced fresh mushrooms to the cooked onions and cook for another two or three minutes. Then steam and chop the broccoli and combine it with the onions and mushrooms in a large baking dish. Cover the top with thinly sliced or grated low-fat mozzarella cheese. Heat before serving until the cheese is completely melted.

Stir-fried vegetables

Stir-fried vegetables can be cooked in a wok or a large skillet. Use defatted stock, water, juice, or wine instead of oil for cooking and stir-fry them only until crisp-tender. It is important to cut the vegetables in approximately the same size pieces for even cooking. Those that take the longest to cook should be placed in the wok or skillet first. Cutting the vegetables diagonally improves the appearance of the finished dish.

Microwave-cooked vegetables

Cover the vegetables to be cooked and follow the time directions for your own oven.

Baked vegetables

The vegetables we usually think of baking are potatoes, sweet potatoes and yams, squash, onions, and eggplant. However, it is possible to bake any kind of vegetable and give it a totally different character than it would have if cooked any other way. You can add greatly to the flavor of a vegetable by baking it in a seasoned fat-free stock, juice, or wine. Seasoned baked vegetables are also good cold.

Baked potatoes are particularly versatile. They are good side dishes and also make wonderful entrées when stuffed with other ingredients. You can stuff them with any kind of food or eat them seasoned only with a little freshly ground black pepper and a sprinkle of Parmesan cheese. They are also delicious served with fat-free gravy, which basically adds no calories or fat to the potato.

I still remember my amazement when James Beard told me about his Overbaked Potato. He bakes it for two hours at 450°. I thought I had misunderstood, but he assured me it was sensational—like a puff pastry shell on the outside, creamy in the middle, and best seasoned only with freshly ground black pepper. I tried it immediately and agreed. It is delicious; however, I like it served not only with freshly ground black pepper but a dash of Parmesan or Romano cheese.

Another great potato dish is the Canyon Ranch Stuft Spud. It is easy to make and a great *JET FUEL* lunch served with a tossed green salad and fresh fruit for dessert. It is even good cold and makes a good brown-bag lunch. Bake two medium potatoes for an hour in a preheated 400° oven. When the potatoes are cool enough to handle, split the tops and remove the pulp, being careful not to tear the skins. Keep the skins warm. Sauté 1 small chopped onion in ¼ cup of defatted chicken stock. Add the potato pulp along with ½ cup of low-fat cottage cheese and 2 tablespoons of Parmesan cheese. Mix well and heat thoroughly. Spoon into the warm potato skins and top with chopped green onion tops.

Baked potatoes can be stuffed with chopped or puréed vegetables; with leftover fish, poultry, or meat; with cheese; or with a combination of all of them. Use your imagination *and* your leftovers!

Baked yams and sweet potatoes

Baked yams and sweet potatoes are fabulous for snacks as well as meals. They are so sweet and satisfying, that they don't need anything on them. It is not possible to improve their wonderful natural taste.

French "fries"

To make French "fries," use a method called oven-frying, which is done without oil. Preheat oven to 375°. Cut baking potatoes into strips— you don't even have to peel them. Spread them on a large nonstick baking sheet or one sprayed with a nonstick spray. Do not overlap. Bake for one hour, turning every 20 minutes. These oven-fried French "fries" are even better than the greasy fast-food variety, *and* whoever has to clean the kitchen will love you.

Broiled vegetables

Broiling vegetables is also an excellent method for cooking them without added fat. Just as we usually don't think of baking many vegetables, most people rarely think of broiling them. You can broil any vegetable either on a broiler rack in the stove or on an outside barbecue grill.

PREPARING INSTANT VEGETABLE SOUPS

In a saucepan, combine defatted stock and cooked vegetables—leftovers are great. Heat, season to taste, and serve. For a thicker soup, purée part of the soup in a blender and pour it back into the remaining soup in the pan.

For a creamy vegetable soup, add nonfat milk instead of stock to your cooked vegetables. Make it just like the instant vegetable soup only don't boil the milk. Bring just to the boiling point.

PREPARING SALADS

Salad does not have to be just a cold combination of lettuce and tomatoes tossed with dressing and served on chilled plates. Warm—or hot-and-cold—salads are exciting. Combining different textures by adding croutons, nuts, and seeds to your salads also adds interest. A salad can be a small, practically calorie-free first course or an entrée.

Here is how to make a wonderful hot-and-cold combination salad. Combine your favorite salad greens as a base. Then slice ½ cup fresh mushrooms for each serving and cook them in *JET FUEL* dressing until they are just tender. Spoon the hot mushroom dressing mixture over each serving. Watch the faces of your guests tak-

ing the first bite. They will be delightfully surprised!

You can do an even more elaborate version
of this salad by sprinkling a little cheese over the
top of each salad before spooning the hot dressing on it and then adding a few toasted nuts over
the top. Your guests will think they are in a
French *nouvelle* restaurant!

Cooking the vegetable in your dressing to
pour over the salad can also be done for practical reasons. If you were planning to use sliced
carrots in a salad but found that they were limp
or tired-looking, just scrape them, slice them
thinly and cook in the dressing until they are
fork-tender and spoon them over the salad. You
will appear to be a culinary genius rather than
someone caught at the last minute with wilted
vegetables.

Salads can also be made with fruits, fish,
poultry, meat, pastas of all kinds, rice, bulgur,
etc. Use your *JET FUEL* Dressing to reduce the
fat content of your salads.

PREPARING LEGUMES (beans and peas)

Wash all dried peas and beans thoroughly before soaking. After washing, soak them in four
times as much water as their volume (for example, eight cups water for two cups of legumes). Remove any of the peas or beans that

float. Soak for several hours or overnight. Slowly bring to a boil in the water in which they were soaked. (Soy beans, however, should be drained and then covered with fresh water.) After the water comes to a boil, reduce the heat and simmer. Cook until tender. Most legumes take about 2 hours to cook, and 1 cup of dried legumes will expand to 2 to 2½ cups during cooking.

PREPARING TOFU (soybean curd)

Tofu basically has no flavor. To add flavor marinate it in *JET FUEL* Dressing, fat-free stock, or fruit juice instead of cooking it in seasoned oils.

PREPARING PASTA

When cooking pasta, remember the Italian guideline *al dente,* which means literally "to the tooth," or slightly resistant to the bite. Overcooking pasta until it is soft and soggy can ruin an otherwise wonderful pasta dish. Pasta should be cooked in a large amount of water. After bringing the water to a boil, add the pasta and allow the water to return to a boil. Reduce the temperature so that the water will not boil over, and cook for about 8 minutes. Some fresh pastas have a much shorter cooking time. Always start testing your pasta after it has cooked 5 or 6 minutes.

You can buy whole wheat pasta and vegetable pasta in health food stores. Also there are pasta shops springing up all over the country where you can buy fresh pastas of all types. You might even enjoy making your own pasta. It's relatively easy and lots of fun. You can make it with or without a pasta machine.

Pasta is versatile and inexpensive. It offers another category of entrées where you can let your imagination run wild. You can combine it with leftovers of all types and it is good hot or cold. There are lots of new pasta cookbooks. It is easy to modify the recipes in them or to modify your own favorites by just reducing or omitting the amount of oil and salt called for and replacing the high-fat ingredients with *JET FUEL* ingredients.

Keep pasta on hand for emergency meals. You can feed lots of people on the spur of the moment with a made-in-minutes pasta meal and look like a super chef.

An example of an easy delicious pasta meal is linguine with clam sauce. Just cook one pound of linguine noodles *al dente,* drain them, toss in a couple of cans of heated undrained chopped clams, and a little grated Parmesan or Romano cheese. If you like a touch of garlic, add a little fresh minced garlic or a sprinkle of garlic powder to the clams before mixing them with the pasta and cheese.

PREPARING DESSERTS

Fresh fruit is the best *JET FUEL* dessert. When you want a special-occasion treat, there are lots of wonderful low-calorie, low-fat, sugar-free dessert books you can use. Read some of them for ideas and then start creating your own.

Puréed fresh fruits make wonderful sauces for other fruits, and can be mixed with nonfat jelled milk (see page 53) and nonfat whipped "cream" (see page 53) topping for interesting desserts of your own.

Make your own fresh-fruit yogurts. Buy plain nonfat or low-fat yogurt without sugar or honey, then add the fresh fruit of your choice and perhaps a little vanilla extract and a dash of cinnamon.

MAKING BEVERAGES

Pilot's Cocktail

You have already read about the virtues of the Pilot's Cocktail and the fact that it not only looks like a drink, but tastes like a drink! It is made with sparkling water such as Perrier or Calistoga —or soda water—a squeeze of fresh lime or lemon juice and a dash of Angostura bitters. You can order a Pilot's Cocktail when you are out as well as making it at home. The ingredients are available in all cocktail lounges.

It is so refreshing, you may find you enjoy

it just as much or even more than any alcoholic beverage, *and* it doesn't contain the calories of alcohol or cause the "double trouble" of alcohol —increasing your appetite and lowering your willpower at the same time. I like my Pilot's Cocktail chilled rather than served over ice, and served in a wineglass garnished with a wedge of lime or lemon.

Milk shakes (and cereal toppings)

JET FUEL milk shakes are delicious, creamy, and naturally refreshing. Freeze the fruit you plan to use in your shake and then combine it with an equal amount of nonfat milk in a blender. My favorite cereal topping is ½ cup of nonfat milk blended together with ½ sliced frozen banana. I like it better than bananas sliced over the cereal, because the taste permeates the whole bowl of cereal.

Melon Coolers

Purée cold diced melon until liquid and serve. You can also add a little Perrier or soda water for a sparkling melon cooler.

Eggnog

For the holidays, surprise your friends with a *JET FUEL* Eggnog. *JET FUEL* Eggnogs are white because you omit the egg yolk for a lower-cholesterol beverage. For one serving, place 1 egg white in a blender and add 1 cup of non-fat milk, 1½ teaspoons fructose, ¾ teaspoon vanilla extract, ¼ teaspoon rum extract, 2 ice cubes and blend until the ice cubes are pulverized and the drink is foamy. Sprinkle with nutmeg.

PREPARING *JET FUEL* SNACKS

Popcorn To pop your corn without oil, use an air popper. If you do not have one, use a heavy iron skillet with a lid and shake it continuously while the corn is popping. A large nonstick saucepan will also serve the purpose.

Tortilla chips Cut corn tortillas into snack size pieces and spread on cookie sheets in a preheated 400° oven for 10 minutes. Turn them over and return to the oven for about 5 more minutes or until they are crisp.

Potato chips Slice peeled baking potatoes as thin as possible (best done with a slicing machine, if you have one). Soak the slices in ice water for about 20 minutes and then drain and pat dry with paper towels. Spread on a nonstick baking sheet without overlapping and bake for fifteen minutes in a preheated 425° oven.

Garbanzo nuts

To make about 3 cups of garbanzo nuts, start with 1½ cups dried garbanzo beans. Put them in a saucepan with enough water to cover them by 3 inches and boil for about 5 minutes. Cover and let stand at room temperature for two hours. Drain, add enough water to again cover by 3 inches, and add one quartered onion and ¼ cup low-sodium soy sauce. Cook about 1 hour or until the beans are tender. Remove the onion, drain well, and spread the beans in a single layer on a nonstick cookie sheet. Sprinkle with onion powder or garlic powder as desired. Bake in a preheated 350° oven, stirring as needed to brown evenly. Continue baking until the beans are brown and crisp, about 50 to 60 minutes.

Croutons

Croutons are wonderful in salads, sprinkled over casseroles, or just eaten as snacks. Making croutons is a wonderful way to use up old bread. Cut the bread slices into ¼-inch squares. Put them on a large cookie sheet and bake in a preheated 350° oven for 20 minutes or until they are a golden brown. Stir frequently so that the squares will brown evenly. If you don't have old bread and still want to make croutons, leave fresh bread slices exposed to the air for several hours to dry them out so they can be cubed easily.

Limited **Fuel Snacks** *Toasted nuts* *and seeds*	To enhance the flavor of raw nuts and seeds so that smaller amounts are adequate, toast them just before using. Place the raw nuts or seeds on a baking sheet in a 350° oven for 8 to 10 minutes, watching carefully because they burn easily. Toasted nuts and seeds are good on salads and on some entrées for both flavor and texture. Their use should be limited because they are high in fat.

MENU PLANNING

If you are planning meals for a family, you might ask, "Is *JET FUEL* all right for children?" It is better than all right—it is *ideal!* In fact, today's children, after having been brought up on *JET FUEL* and exercise, will have naturally acquired the bodies their parents struggled to shape.

JET FUEL meal planning is the reverse of traditional meal planning. You don't plan a chicken dinner. You plan to have chicken *with* dinner. It is amazing how much difference this shift in thinking will make in the creation of your future menus.

When planning your weekly menus, consider your time. Prepare as many dishes in advance as possible. Always build in a couple of "catch-up" meals. That is when you use every-thing you might have left over from the two or three previous days. The French turn leftovers into a superchic dish by mix-ing them with cooked white beans and calling it a cassoulet. You can do the same thing with your leftovers, using either the same white beans or other kinds of legumes, pasta, or rice—and dreaming up your own name for it.

For breakfast, dare to be different. The classic American breakfast of bacon and eggs should be history. Unfortunately it is still the daily fare for millions of ordinary people. For millions more, each day begins with a sweet roll or a couple of doughnuts and a cup of coffee. And of course, there are those who try to start the day without any fuel intake at all. This group always reminds me of my favorite cartoon, which has a picture of a fat, unpleasant-looking man with the cap-tion *People who try to lose weight by skipping breakfast end up fat and mean!*

Most "diet book" menu plans give you one breakfast for an entire week and then just say "Repeat." I get bored with the same thing every morning, so I have given you seven different ideas to get your day started. Use your imagination and come up with some breakfast ideas of your own. Dare to experiment *and* be different!

DAY 1

Breakfast
Fresh fruit
Whole wheat bagel or English muffin, toasted
   with your own favorite low-fat cheese such
   as ricotta, mozzarella, or cottage cheese
   (*Try topping it off with a little of the fruit.
   It's delicious!*)

Lunch
Tuna sandwich
(Try making it with water-packed tuna on whole wheat bread, just enough mayonnaise for moisture and flavor, lettuce, sliced tomatoes, and a sprinkle of freshly ground black pepper.)
Relish tray of carrot and celery sticks
Fresh fruit

Dinner
Citrus salad
(lettuce with diced orange and grapefruit and with JET FUEL Dressing with cumin)
Chicken—without the skin
Brown rice
Green and yellow vegetables
Fruit yogurt
(Combine plain nonfat or low-fat yogurt with diced fresh fruit.)

Snack
Cereal with nonfat milk
(If you eat a late dinner, have your daily snack in the late afternoon around four o'clock. If you eat an early dinner, save your snack for later in the evening, around eight o'clock. This will keep you from getting hungry and eating inferior fuel snacks just because they are available. If you won't be at home, take portable snacks with you. Some of the snacks I am suggesting can be easily carried with you. Others are more practically eaten at home. Dried fruit is always a handy snack to keep in your desk drawer or the glove compartment of your car.)

DAY 2

Breakfast
Grape-Nuts with fresh fruit and nonfat milk.
Lunch
Lettuce, chicken, and cheese salad with hot mushroom dressing (see page 64).
Whole wheat toast
Broiled grapefruit
Dinner
Sliced tomatoes
Pasta Primavera
(Combine the cooked pasta with defatted chicken stock thickened with cornstarch and seasoned with Parmesan or Romano cheese. Add a colorful assortment of cooked crisp vegetables cut in bite-size pieces and toss thoroughly.)
Melon
Snack
Fruit and yogurt

DAY 3

Breakfast
Danish Rye Cereal with part-skim ricotta cheese
(To make Danish Rye Cereal, combine 1 cup unprocessed rye berries, 2 teaspoons ground cinnamon, 1 teaspoon caraway seeds, 1 tablespoon vanilla extract, and 3 cups water in a saucepan. Mix well and bring to a boil. Reduce the heat and cook, covered, for 1 hour, stirring occasionally and adding more water if necessary to prevent scorching. During the last 15 minutes of cooking time, add 1/4 cup

raisins. Serve with a little part-skim ricotta cheese on the top of the hot cereal. It tastes like a Danish pastry. This cereal is also good cold and can be stored in the freezer for fast future breakfasts. Makes 2½ cups.)

Lunch

Fresh fruit salad with Banana Yogurt Dressing
(Combine diced oranges and diced fresh pineapple or drained pineapple chunks packed in their own juice and a diced red apple. Combine a cup of nonfat or low-fat yogurt in a blender with a sliced banana and pour over the top for dressing. This is colorful and delicious.)

Bran muffins

Dinner

Marinated vegetable salad
(Marinate colorful assorted cooked cold vegetables in JET FUEL Dressing and serve over lettuce.)

Poached Salmon with Dill Sauce
(To make Dill Sauce, combine a cup of nonfat or low-fat yogurt, 1 teaspoon of crushed tarragon, and 2 teaspoons of crushed dillweed. Add a dash of salt and mix thoroughly. The sauce is best if it is prepared the day before you plan to use it.)

Baked potato

Steamed cucumbers

Fresh berries

Snack

Whole wheat breadsticks with low-fat mozzarella cheese

DAY 4

Breakfast

Shredded wheat with banana-milk topping
(Combine ½ cup nonfat milk and ½ sliced banana in a blender. Frozen banana slices make a thicker, creamier topping.)

Lunch

Tostada
(To make the tostada, start with a whole toasted tortilla or toasted tortilla chips [see page 70]. Cover with finely chopped lettuce, diced tomatoes, chopped onion if desired, and a little JET FUEL Dressing with cumin. Add a little cooked chopped chicken or turkey and grated cheese. Use green Ortega chile strips for garnish. Top with Mexican salsa and a dollop of sour cream.)

Mexican fruit plate
(All fruits grow somewhere in Mexico—so any fruit combination is a Mexican fruit plate!)

Dinner

Chow Mein over Chinese Noodles
(To make fat-free toasted Chinese noodles, break whole wheat spaghetti into 2-inch pieces. Cover with water and boil about 12 minutes. Drain thoroughly and spread evenly in a large baking dish. Bake for 1 hour in a preheated 375° oven, turning frequently to toast evenly. If you use 4 ounces of whole wheat pasta, it makes about 4 cups of noodles. Make the sauce by combining 2 tablespoons low-sodium soy sauce, a heaping tablespoon cornstarch, 2 tablespoons rice vinegar, 2

teaspoons fructose and mixing until the
cornstarch is completely dissolved. Add 1
cup water, place over low heat, and stir
until the sauce is slightly thickened. Stir-fry
a combination of thinly sliced celery,
without leaves, bell pepper, fresh
mushrooms, onions, Chinese cabbage, and
water chestnuts. Add pea pods and bean
sprouts and cook until just crisp-tender.
Mix with the sauce and serve over the
Chinese noodles. Makes 4 servings.)
Papaya with lime

Snack

Pumpernickel bagel topped with your
favorite low-fat cheese
(Or make JET FUEL sandwich spread.
Combine 1 cup of part-skim ricotta cheese
and 2 tablespoons low-fat plain yogurt in a
food processor or a blender and whip until
completely smooth. Store, covered, in
refrigerator. It's also wonderful on toast for
breakfast.)

DAY 5

Breakfast

Fresh fruit
Cinnamon-Cheese Toast
(Spread whole wheat toast with your
favorite low-fat cheese or JET FUEL
sandwich spread and sprinkle with ground
cinnamon. Place the toast under the broiler
until the cheese is hot.)

Lunch
Fresh vegetable salad with *JET FUEL* Italian
    Dressing (see pages 51-52)
Linguine with clam sauce (see page 67)
Orange and grapefruit sections

Dinner
Cole slaw
Roast turkey with fat-free gravy (see page 50)
Baked sweet potato
Vegetable medley
    *(a colorful combination of steamed
    vegetables)*
Baked bananas
    *(Split the bananas lengthwise and put them
    in a pan or baking dish, cut side up.
    Sprinkle with ground cinnamon and place
    under the broiler until lightly browned.)*

Snack
Cereal with nonfat milk

DAY 6

Breakfast
Grapefruit
Mexican Scrambled Eggs
    *(Combine 1 egg with 1 egg white. Add
    chopped tomato, onion, canned green
    chile, a dash of ground cumin, and a dash
    of chili powder and cook, stirring
    constantly, in a nonstick pan.)*
Hot corn tortillas

Lunch
Chef's Salad (otherwise known as Clean the
    Refrigerator)

(Combine raw vegetables, leftover turkey, chicken, or meat, and low-fat mozzarella cheese cut in thin strips with lettuce and sprouts. Serve with JET FUEL Dressing.)
Toasted pumpernickel bagel
Melon

Dinner

Marinated Eggplant Antipasto
(Peel 1 eggplant and slice horizontally into ½-inch slices. Steam 5 minutes or until just done and place in a glass baking dish. Cover the top with finely chopped tomato, onion, and parsley. Pour JET FUEL Dressing with cumin in it over the top. Cover and refrigerate until cold. Serve on lettuce leaves. Chances are, your guests won't know what they're eating—but they'll love it. Makes 4 servings.)

Spaghetti
(Cook whole wheat spaghetti and toss with a fat-free spaghetti sauce—your own favorite recipe, omitting the oil—and sprinkle with Parmesan or Romano cheese.)

Frozen grapes (It takes longer to eat them!)
(Leave fresh grapes in the freezer until they are hard. These also make great snacks for children.)

Snack

Apple and low-fat cheese

DAY 7

Breakfast

Baked apple with vanilla yogurt
(*Make your own vanilla yogurt by adding a little vanilla extract to plain nonfat or low-fat yogurt. It's also good with a little ground cinnamon.*)
Bran muffin

Lunch

Pita bread sandwich
(*Combine grated carrot, shredded lettuce, diced tomatoes, alfalfa sprouts, and grated low-fat cheese and stuff into a pita pocket. Combine nonfat or low-fat yogurt with a little JET FUEL Dressing and spoon over the filling.*)
Fresh fruit

Dinner

Egg drop soup (see page 50)
Teriyaki Flank Steak
(*Combine ½ cup low-sodium soy sauce, 1 can frozen concentrated pineapple juice, 2 buds garlic, crushed, 1 tablespoon fresh peeled, grated ginger root or ½ teaspoon powdered ginger. It is better to make your marinade the day before. Marinate the flank steak for 1 to 2 hours before cooking. Broil 3 to 5 minutes on each side, depending upon the thickness of the meat, for a rare steak.*)
Brown rice
Stir-fried pea pods and water chestnuts
Pineapple with coconut sauce
(*To make coconut sauce, combine 1 cup nonfat jelled milk [see page 53] with ¾ teaspoon vanilla extract and ¾ teaspoon*

coconut extract and blend until creamy.
Pour over the pineapple. It tastes like a
piña colada!)
Snack
Cereal with nonfat milk

SERVING SUGGESTIONS

If a picture is worth a thousand words, a meal that is beautifully and imaginatively presented can be worth as much as many hours spent in preparation and cooking.

Successful food presentation does not need to be time-consuming nor require a course in garniture from a culinary institute. Just learning to cut vegetables in different and unusual ways adds a creative touch to your raw vegetable plates and salads. It also makes your cooked vegetables more attractive. For example, the next time you are cutting a carrot, try cutting it on the diagonal instead of just straight across. If you really want to impress your friends, make carrot flowers. There are several good books available about garniture. However, just a plate of colorful raw or cold cooked vegetables, such as broccoli florets, radishes, carrots, jicama, cherry tomatoes, or cauliflower florets arranged on a bed of curly lettuce leaves and garnished with sprigs of parsley can look like a photo on the cover of *Gourmet* magazine.

Serving meals in courses also makes the menu seem more special *and* it slows down your eating time, so that you are satisfied with less food.

Other tips for eating more slowly include using a three-tined instead of a four-tined fork, teaspoons instead of soup spoons for soup, demitasse spoons instead of teaspoons for dessert, and chopsticks.

To make less food look like more, use smaller-size plates

and bowls and smaller glasses. Also slicing fish, poultry, or meat very thinly will make a three- or four-ounce serving look like a lot more than that.

ENTERTAINING

As a high performance person you may be living exclusively on *JET FUEL*, but the minute you have company for dinner, your whole concept of fuel changes. You are afraid of serving company *JET FUEL* for dinner for fear of disappointing them. You feel you have to start with rich inferior fuel for hors d'oeuvres. Then you pour heavy Roquefort dressing over their salads, adding just as much fat as possible—and then you serve a prime steak for the entrée.

Your own dessert on a daily basis may be sliced fresh fruit, but for company you probably will consider stopping at a bakery for gooey pastries. In fact, the more important the company, the harder you try to destroy them.

Plan your next dinner party as though you were going to be the guest. You will be amazed how differently your planning will progress *and* how much more your guests will appreciate the experience. Remember Oscar Wilde's great line: "I have the simplest of tastes—I am always satisfied with the best." *JET FUEL is* the best!

You don't have to give up holiday goodies or special-occasion treats—just keep the *JET FUEL* mix in the proper proportions. Also, remember that you don't have to drink a quart of eggnog or eat a whole birthday cake to enjoy either the treat or the experience. Remember moderation and common sense!

Jet Fuel in Motion

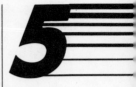

In Restaurants, on Jets, Brown-Bagging, and Being a Guest

Weight-loss programs promoting prepackaged meals, pills, powdered mixes, or set menus get in the way of your life-style. Even stay-fit programs with very rigid dietary guidelines were never designed for high-performance people who don't want to miss anything.

Not only are these programs difficult to follow whenever you are eating away from home, they are virtually impossible to follow when traveling, dining out in restaurants, or going to other people's dinner parties. Can you imagine going to a restaurant and drinking your dinner while everyone else is eating "real food"?

Wouldn't you rather sit with your friends in a candlelit Italian restaurant enjoying a big salad with the dressing served on the side, then having a plate of linguine with seafood, seasoned with a little freshly ground Parmesan cheese and a bowl of fresh berries for dessert—knowing this is a *JET FUEL* dinner?

EATING IN RESTAURANTS

Eating in a restaurant is not only an enjoyable event but a way of life for many high-performance people.

Most restaurants serve portions seemingly designed for people well over six feet tall and weighing more than two hundred pounds. Therefore—unless you fit this description —if you eat everything you are served routinely, your weight is going to start climbing.

I will share a little-known secret with you! I have eaten in restaurants of all types all over the world, and I have never yet been in one where they forced me to eat everything I was served. Therefore, I think you can safely assume that you are never going to be forced to clean your plate either. Also, remember when you are dining out in a lovely restaurant that you are there for the total experience, not just the food.

Order your fish, poultry, or meat broiled, baked, or poached without sauce and your salad without dressing. Always ask for your sauces and salad dressings on the side. By doing this you do not miss the opportunity of tasting a particularly delicious sauce or salad dressing but you do control the amount you eat. Don't let this decision be made for you by someone in the kitchen.

You will be pleasantly surprised to find how very little salad dressing or sauce it takes to add significantly to the flavor and moisture of your salads, vegetables, and entrées.

When you are trying to use less fat for fuel, why put butter on your bread? Butter or margarine in no way represent the creativity of a talented chef. They are just plain fat. When you are purposely adding fat to your fuel mix, use it to experience the sauces and salad dressings, which may be memorable.

JET FUEL is available in practically all restaurants, and you are in control because you are the one ordering the food.

In ethnic restaurants where you may not be familiar with the dishes, ask your waiter or waitress to explain them to you.

Now that you know the guidelines, just do the best you can. Improper fueling once in a while is certainly better than continual consumption of low-quality fuel.

FLYING ON JETS

JET FUEL on airplanes prevents jet lag!

There is a simple four-step program involved:

1. Don't drink any alcoholic beverages.
2. Don't eat any high-fat foods.
3. Don't overeat.
4. *Do* drink lots of water all during the flight.

Avoiding alcoholic beverages is important because you are not pressurized to ground level, but to around 5,000 feet. Therefore the effects of alcohol are much more pronounced. What many people refer to as jet lag is really nothing more than an airborne hangover.

I actually have had people tell me that they couldn't possibly not drink at least a little wine with dinner because they were flying first class, and it seemed dumb not to take advantage of the free drinks. My question is always "How much more is it costing you to fly first class?" The difference is usually enormous—and just how much can you drink? Be realistic—the advantage of first-class flying is a larger seat, more leg room, and more personal service—*not* free booze!

Always carry a small bottle of Angostura bitters with you and make your own Pilot's Cocktails.

Avoiding rich fatty foods is important because the fat

temporarily inhibits the free flow of oxygen-carrying corpuscles to the brain and robs you of energy, making you feel tired.

In order to have *JET FUEL* meals while flying it is usually necessary to order them at least twenty-four hours before your departure time. Almost all airlines have special meals available at no extra charge. Two good selections include a cold seafood plate and a fresh fruit and cottage cheese salad. There is also a low-calorie meal available on some airlines that includes a salad, broiled fish, and a piece of fresh fruit for dessert. Simply eating too much will also make you more uncomfortable than it would at ground level.

If you can't order a special meal—or your special meal is not boarded—then just apply the *JET FUEL* guidelines to what is available. Don't eat the nuts; don't butter the bread; don't use the salad dressing; scrape the sauce off of the entrée; and leave the airline cake on the tray.

Drinking lots of water is important to prevent dehydration caused by the reduced oxygen in the pressurized cabin. Drink at least one eight-ounce glass of water every hour. Pilot's Cocktails do count as part of your water intake, so they play a double role, substituting for both your drinks and your water.

By sticking to *JET FUEL,* you will not only avoid jet lag, you will arrive happy and energized from the flight. Where else can you find time without outside interruptions such as the telephone, meetings, and emergencies? It is a wonderful opportunity to plan and arrange your work schedule or just relax and enjoy a good book. You may find that the *JET FUEL* approach to flying actually enables you to arrive more relaxed with an even more positive attitude than you had on boarding—a real "happy landing"!

HOTELS AND MOTELS

Another problem for the frequent traveler is the unfortunate fact that most hotels do not offer nonfat milk or low-fat dairy products. A simple solution is to find a nearby market or deli and buy your own milk, yogurt, cottage cheese, or whatever. If there is not a refrigerator in your room, ask the manager to keep these foods in the hotel's refrigerator for you. Remember —you are the guest.

This same solution works beautifully for fresh fruit in season, which is often not found on hotel menus. Not only are you in control of your own fuel intake, but you are spending less money for higher-quality fuel.

JET FUEL IN A BROWN BAG

JET FUEL is far more practical for portable meals than ordinary fuel.

Whole-grain breads have a firmer texture than refined white breads, so sandwiches stay fresher-looking and -tasting for a longer period of time. Also, using less butter, margarine, or mayonnaise on sandwiches helps keep them from getting soggy.

Raw vegetables and fresh whole fruits are easily packed to go as are small cartons of low-fat cottage cheese and yogurt.

Throw in a bottle of Perrier, a small bottle of Angostura bitters, and a wedge of lemon or lime, and you can even enjoy a Pilot's Cocktail with your lunch!

Dried fruits make marvelous snacks to carry with you in a handbag or briefcase or to keep in your desk or car.

Brown bag lunches that used to get chuckles at the office are moving into the status stratum and are considered a first-class fueling technique for high performers on the job.

Over thirty-four million workers in the United States

carry lunch to work each day *and* recent research shows that families who brown-bag tend to have more money and are better educated than those who don't.

Packing your lunch not only saves you money but gives you extra time for other activities, such as walking and writing personal letters. It also allows you to control the quality and quantity of your meal.

With the rising popularity of the portable meal (in 1982 forty-six billion dollars were spent on ingredients), manufacturers are coming out with many new convenience products. A good example is the cold box—a plastic container with a freezable lid—that will keep contents cold for up to five hours. The smallest size will hold one or two sandwiches and fits easily into a briefcase. Larger sizes are available for larger meals.

BEING A GUEST

When you are a guest for a meal in someone else's house, you face the greatest problem the high-performance person ever experiences in trying to stick to *JET FUEL*. Your host or hostess may have the same overindulgent attitude discussed earlier. He or she will try to make you feel guilty about not finishing some high-fat sauce-laden dish with statements like "I made it myself" or even worse "I made it just for you." In this situation you might explain "I am allergic to fat. It keeps my clothes from fitting."

When you are going to be a guest in someone else's home for several days, *plan ahead*. If you know that your Aunt Bertha does not have anything remotely resembling *JET FUEL* in her house, surprise her! Arrive with a lovely decorated basket of all the things *you* want—just don't tell her that it is really your own survival kit.

It is important to remember that you are never a victim.

You are always in control. You are in the pilot's seat!

It is possible for you to eat in the most exceptional restaurants, pampering yourself by ordering the most scrumptious dishes the chef can create for you, entertain with such style and imagination that your reputation as a host or hostess is impressive—and do it *all* on *JET FUEL!*

Jet Age Psychology

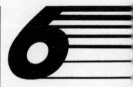

So many people truly don't know what it is like to really feel good. They have been trudging along on ordinary and inferior fuel for so long that they think the way they feel is "normal."

If you are in this category, prepare yourself for takeoff, because after a week on *JET FUEL* you are going to experience a new natural high that is so fabulous, you may well wonder what is wrong with you. Actually everything is right with you. So enjoy your newfound energy and fantastic feeling of self-esteem.

This feeling is addictive. You will never be able to give it up permanently now that you have experienced it.

If you blow it, don't feel guilty. Feel human.

We all learn from our mistakes. Even if you've taken a crash landing, don't berate yourself. You already feel miserable enough. The only way to take off again is to get right back on *JET FUEL.*

Compulsively jumping on the scales every morning and letting the numbers you read dictate your mood for the day is decidedly not the way to manage your eating behavior. You never judge other people by the numbers, so why judge yourself that way?

Can you imagine seeing an attractive woman walking across a room and thinking, Great figure—about 125 pounds? Of course not. We all judge other peoples' bodies by the way they look. So why not apply this same principle to our own bodies?

If weighing yourself every day served any useful purpose, it would be different; but in fact, it is counterproductive. You do not take into account the normal fluctuations in body fluids that affect your weight on a daily basis.

You are trying to lose weight only to find that you have gained two pounds, and guess what happens to your behavior? You are discouraged and unhappy with yourself, so you eat more all day long. Conversely if your scale weight is less than you expected it to be, you are so delighted with yourself that you eat much less than you normally would during the day.

Another problem with scale weight is that it does not tell you what percentage of your weight is muscle and what percentage is fat. The higher percentage of muscle you have relative to the percentage of fat, the better your metabolism is; and the better your metabolism is, the more calories you burn up every day. Therefore, a higher metabolism means that you can take in more fuel every day and still maintain your desired weight.

Instead of jumping on the scales, stand stark naked in front of a full-length mirror. This will tell you how you really look. If you want to keep a record of the progress you are making in the pursuit of a better body, do it with a tape measure—not a scale.

The combination of *JET FUEL* and adequate exercise is burning up your excess fat and building muscle tissue.

Muscle tissue weighs more than fat; therefore even though you look slimmer and feel more fit, you may not weigh much less on a scale; so look in the mirror, measure yourself, and *smile!*

Never skip breakfast just because you had too much to eat the night before. It's a crutch used by many compulsive night eaters, and it does not work.

Statistics show that a staggering number of Americans—roughly 35 to 45 percent—routinely skip the most important meal of the day. Just as its name indicates, you are breaking the fast of the night, and you need the early-morning nourishment to produce enough energy to keep you going through the morning. Numerous studies demonstrate that workers who skip breakfast become less efficient in the late-morning hours, as do students, who have trouble concentrating on their studies.

In fact, skipping meals prevents effective weight management. Each time you eat, your metabolism is raised and you burn up the calories much faster. Therefore, it is better to have three smaller meals and a snack if necessary rather than one or two large meals. Your metabolism will hum along at a higher rate, burning up the calories you are taking in more efficiently.

Stop eating when you are no longer hungry. If you continue to eat until you have that bloated, uncomfortable feeling associated with being too full, you will be almost certain to go on overeating. This is because you started feeling guilty and out of control rather than proud of yourself. Guilt is the fuel that runs the overeating machine!

Also, you are more likely to become a garbage eater. What is garbage? Garbage is food that is left on other people's plates. Garbage belongs in the garbage disposal—not in you! It will end up in the same place whether you put it directly in the disposal or first process it through you. You will look better and feel better if the disposal gets it first.

For some strange reason that behavioral psychologists have never been able to explain, it is this feeling of discomfort from overeating that often triggers a binge of compulsive eating. You are more likely to come home and raid the refrigerator when you are already uncomfortably full than if you had declined dessert because you were no longer hungry. When you are proud of yourself, you are *in control.*

It is important to remember this when teaching good eating habits to children. Never suggest they finish everything on their plates because of all the poor, starving children somewhere. Don't tell them that they can't have dessert unless they finish everything on their plates. When dessert is held out as a reward for eating everything else, most children are certainly not going to give up the reward of dessert even though they are uncomfortably full. They feel they have earned it, and therefore are somehow going to stuff it in. This same attitude learned in childhood is displayed by adults when they are too full to enjoy dessert but not about to miss having something special. How many times have you been in a restaurant with a friend who said after the meal "I am so full, I shouldn't have finished that sandwich." Then the waiter arrives and asks if you would like to order dessert, and your friend, instead of telling the waiter "No, thank you," asks "What is it?" Isn't this a perfect example of programmed response?

A good way to reinforce the concept of not overeating is to plan to exercise about thirty minutes after each meal. Stop eating while you still feel like doing some form of physical activity. Another positive result of exercising after meals is that the elevated metabolic rate that is always caused by eating is further raised by exercising. You know that the positive advantages of increased metabolism are maintained for many hours afterward.

Any form of exercise will do. Go for a walk, take a bicycle ride, play tennis, swim, dance, or make love. The important thing is to do something besides just sit and get fat.

The more slowly you eat, the smaller amount of food it

takes to satisfy your appetite. The brain can't tell you that you aren't hungry anymore until the blood sugar has risen sufficiently to trigger brain response. If you are wolfing your food down as fast as you can, you may literally be too full *before you know it!*

There are many classic behavioral suggestions for slowing the rate at which you consume food. Some of them were already mentioned in the chapter on serving suggestions, such as dividing meals into several courses; using a three-tined instead of a four-tined fork; using smaller spoons for such things as soups, cereals, and desserts; and of course, using chopsticks, which are particularly effective if you don't know how to use them well! There are many others, among which are: eating consciously by enjoying each bite to its fullest, chewing each bite a prescribed number of times, and putting your fork down between bites. Don't combine eating with any other activities such as watching television, reading, or playing cards. I am sure you have heard most of them. They all work for different people at different times. My advice is to use any or all of them which help you.

Food should be a concern, not an obsession.

Simply saying "I *will* fly on *JET FUEL*" instead of "I wish" makes all the difference in the world to your success.

JET FUEL is a strategy of winning with food. Remember —anytime you are going to eat or drink anything, ask yourself, "Is my eating behavior helping me to achieve my goals? Is it *JET FUEL?*"

Visualize yourself constantly as the stronger, smarter, and slimmer person you are becoming. Enjoy sitting straighter, standing taller, and walking more briskly.

You are taking more interest in your clothes because you know you look better.

Your sex life is improving because the better shape you are in, the more sensuous you feel. Now that you're proud of your body, you don't have to make love in the dark!

You are achieving more success professionally because you are making better decisions more rapidly.

You are experiencing that wonderfully exuberant feeling of fulfillment in every facet of your life.

You are a winner—you are flying on *JET FUEL!*

ABOUT THE AUTHOR

Author of twelve books, Jeanne Jones leads an active and exciting life. She is one of the leading writers, lecturers, and consultants in the nutrition field. Entertaining with flair and imagination all over the world has gained for her an international reputation as a hostess. Her home is in La Jolla, California.